Fascial Release *for* Structural Balance

James Earls & Thomas Myers

Lotus Publishing
Chichester, England

North Atlantic Books
Berkeley, California

First published in 2010 by
Lotus Publishing
Apple Tree Cottage, Inlands Road, Nutbourne, Chichester, PO18 8RJ and
North Atlantic Books
P O Box 12327
Berkeley, California 94712

Anatomical Drawings Amanda Williams
Text and Cover Design Wendy Craig
Printed and Bound in the UK by Scotprint

Fascial Release for Structural Balance is sponsored by the Society for the Study of Native Arts and Sciences, a nonprofit educational corporation whose goals are to develop an educational and crosscultural perspective linking various scientific, social, and artistic fields; to nurture a holistic view of arts, sciences, humanities, and healing; and to publish and distribute literature on the relationship of mind, body, and nature.

The Publisher has made every effort to trace holders of copyright in original material and to seek permission for its use in *Fascial Release for Structural Balance*. Should this have proved impossible, copyright holders are asked to contact the Publisher so that suitable acknowledgment can be made at the first opportunity.

In memory of Stephen Stevenson, a friend, a colleague.
With my sincere thanks to his family for permission to use his images within this book.

British Library Cataloguing-in-Publication Data
A CIP record for this book is available from the British Library
ISBN 978 1 905367 18 4 (Lotus Publishing)
ISBN 978 1 55643 937 7 (North Atlantic Books)

Library of Congress Cataloguing-in-Publication Data
Earls, James.
Fascial release for structural balance / James Earls and Tom Myers.
        p. ; cm.
    Includes bibliographical references and index.
    Summary: "Fascial release for structural balance is a fully illustrated
introductory guide to structural anatomy and fascial release
therapy"--Provided by publisher.
    ISBN 978-1-905367-18-4 (Lotus Pub.) -- ISBN 978-1-55643-937-7 (North Atlantic Books)
            1. Manipulation (Therapeutics) 2. Myofascial pain syndromes. 3. Fasciae (Anatomy) I. Myers,
            Thomas W., LMT. II. Title.
    [DNLM: 1. Fascia--anatomy & histology. 2. Massage--methods. 3. Musculoskeletal
Manipulations--methods. WE 500 E12f 2010]
    RM724.E17 2010
    615.8'2--dc22
                                    2010014999

Contents

Introduction/How to Use This Book

Each person's structural pattern is unique – an expression of the many variables that combine to create the shape in each of us. Thus any analysis of structure is necessarily limited. Whether by conscious or unconscious choice, by inherited design or learnt habit, through physical or psychological trauma, we shape our body and therefore the tissue that supports it into one of the six billion possibilities that is you or your client. To cover each and every of the possible vagaries of shape would require a tome many times larger than this one.

In this book we have therefore guided you to see many of the common tendencies, with visual examples where possible. Each chapter gives you an introduction to the structural anatomy of a portion of the body, followed by hints and ideas on what to look for when analyzing clients, rounded off with strategies and tools to address the fascial sheets and guy ropes within it.

Due to the holistic nature of human patterning, it is difficult to give a linear and methodical analysis of each and every possibility, and it would bore the reader to do so. Where the logic behind a technique was not clearly covered within the anatomical or BodyReading introduction, we have given structural examples alongside the technique.

In some cases only one example is given, as it would again tire the reader to be constantly reminded that 'if the opposite pattern is present then the tissue relationship will be reversed'. A simple understanding of the antagonistic relationship of muscles is presumed. Although this book can stand alone, many of the techniques presented here draw on the Anatomy Trains theory set forth in *Anatomy Trains: Myofascial Meridians for Manual and Movement Therapists* (Myers 2009), and we have not repeated all of the detail of each Anatomy Train. That information is readily available in other sources should you wish to research it further, though a summary of each is given in the appendix for easy reference. Nevertheless, readers unfamiliar with 'Anatomy Trains' will still find in this manual many of the necessary tools and much of the understanding needed to start making changes with their clients' structures.

The techniques are given in a roughly anatomical sequence rather than according to the Anatomy Trains theory; though where the target area does belong within the territory of a Train it is referenced for your convenience. This allows the practitioner to take advantage of the fascial continuities by extending the release of one area by working on adjacent elements of the same line. So, for example, if the hamstrings seem reluctant to release or lengthen, then following the Superficial Back Line of which they are a significant element we may achieve further release by working with the gastrocnemius or sacrotuberous ligament. A key for the abbreviations of the lines is given at the end of this section.

BodyReading does take practice and we have a number of other resources to help you with it should you wish to take it further; for more details, see Resources. Likewise, we run a number of workshops throughout the world in which we combine the Anatomy Trains theory, BodyReading, and Fascial Release Technique (FRT).

The techniques that are listed are not complete. Certain areas have been omitted because their intimacy or their delicate nature does not lend itself to learning without the practical guidance available in a workshop or mentoring relationship. These techniques can be creatively adapted to individual patterns in terms of direction, depth, and choice of your body position and applicator tool used – fingers, palm, knuckles or elbow. What is important is your understanding of what you are trying to achieve and the nature of the tissue you are working with. Much of this will depend on palpatory feedback, something that can be learnt only through practice and with a certain amount of guidance. But the reflective practitioner will be well equipped to face a wide range of clients with confidence after working through the many aspects of this book. We hope to encourage the reader to see the techniques as templates and ideas that are malleable to fit the needs of the client and their individual tissue. Working with the idea of each intervention being a 'communication between two intelligent systems' and achieving and maintaining the lock in the tissue are two of the most important elements of this approach. We therefore recommend even the seasoned practitioner to spend time with the introductory sections of the book.

Most anatomy taught today uses the traditional elements of the body, generally ignoring the important qualities of the fascial webbing and, in particular, the myofascia which this book addresses. Using the names of individual muscles can give the impression that they are discrete, separate entities in their own right, but several lines of current research are showing the limitations of this way of thinking (Myers 2009, Huijing 2008, Stecco 2009, Van der Wal 2009). In order to describe the mechanics of each of the techniques within this book we have used familiar muscular terminology. But each time we name a muscle we hope to bring to mind the idea of continuous sheaths and planes of strong elastic tissue in which are contained the contractile elements that we call muscles. When we refer to any muscle within this text, please realise that we consider it to have wider connection in the body beyond its traditional origin and insertion.

Our main aim is to encourage you to think and analyze in a different way: rather than being drawn by the client's story of their pain, look further afield and build a story of their structure, work with them to explore it, develop an alternative strategy and experiment with a structural approach using fascial release. This book provides an introduction to this exciting and rewarding approach to bodywork. We encourage you to take it further by attending any of the increasing number of workshops available worldwide. We look forward to meeting you in person one day soon.

We wish you every success.

Thomas Myers & James Earls

Key to Anatomy Trains Abbreviations

SFL – Superficial Front Line

SBL – Superficial Back Line

LTL – Lateral Line

SPL – Spiral Line

DFL – Deep Front Line

SFAL – Superficial Front Arm Line

DFAL – Deep Front Arm Line

SBAL – Superficial Back Arm Line

DBAL – Deep Back Arm Line

FFL – Front Functional Line

BFL – Back Functional Line

An Introduction to Fascial Release Technique

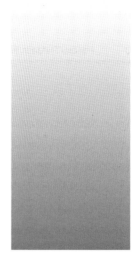

1

Human Patterning

All therapists of whatever method, but especially manual therapists, are seeking greater order in human movement patterning, making forays into the porous border between structure and function. Any change of behavior is a change of movement. But for sustained change in the postural basis of movement, attention to the fascial tissues and their properties is essential.

Every tangible structure in the real world is a compromise between the need for stability – necessary to maintain a coherent structure so that repetitive processes can happen easily and reliably – and mobility, which allows the structure to deal with all kinds of environmental novelty responsively and without 'breaking' essential parts.

While banks and mountains lie at the stability end of the spectrum, living creatures tend to lean toward the mobility end. Plants, mostly anchored, have settled on fiber made from the carbohydrate cellulose as their main structural element. Large land animals, including humans, primarily use the pliable protein collagen fiber for creating structures that are stable enough to be physiologically viable and at the same time thoroughly mobile in their ability to move through the environment and manipulate it to their own ends.

Thus, a thorough familiarity with the properties and positioning of collagenous tissue – which makes up most of the tendons, ligaments, aponeuroses, muscle envelopes, organ bags and attachments, and sheets of biological fabric – is vital to successful manual therapy and physical training. Understanding muscles and nerves – though essential – is not enough. Approaching the fascia requires a different eye, a different touch, and tissue-specific techniques.

This stability/mobility compromise can lead to 'compromising' situations at both ends of the spectrum. On the stability end, parts that should stay mobile relative to other parts can become fascially or neurologically stuck together and unable to move differentially. This results in congestion and mechanical strain locally, or additional loading in linked – but sometimes quite distant – 'elsewheres' (figure 1.1).

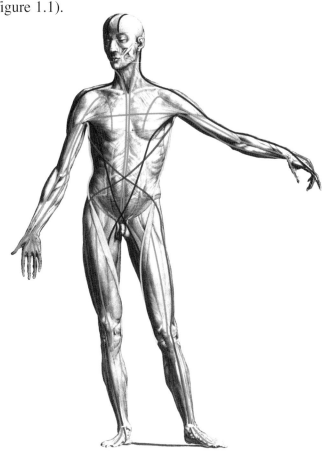

Figure 1.1: The Anatomy Trains Myofascial Meridians constitute one map of how compensation can be shifted from one part of the body to another, quite distant part.

On the other side, sometimes parts that should stay closely bound become too movable relative to each other, and this hypermobility can cause friction (and thus inflammation and its aftermath). This excess movement also necessitates either muscular or fascial compensation (read: contraction or binding) somewhere else to create enough stability for function (like walking, standing, sitting, work or sport) to continue without breaking down.

Muscle 'knots', spasms, long-term tension in trigger points, less-than-efficient movement patterns, thickened or glued fascia, 'dead' areas of sensori-motor amnesia and, of course, tissue pain are all ultimately sequelae of the body's attempt to deal with these stability/mobility issues as best it can under the available circumstances.

So, as therapists seeking to restore structural integrity and balance for our clients, we address ourselves every day to this complex array of adaptations in the 'neuro-myofascial' web. Welcome to a practical guide to negotiating these patterns via manipulative interventions in the highly innervated muscle and connective tissues.

In this book we concentrate especially on the fascial/connective tissue part of this patterning troika. Everyone knows their muscles and bones, and much study has gone into them. The connective tissues that mediate between the two have received less focus and are thus less well understood. It is to the properties and disposition of these adaptable tissues that we now turn our attention.

One caveat: Any linear presentation, e.g. this book, must necessarily present the approach in terms of individually named 'parts', but the challenge for any therapist is to assemble such piecemeal 'techniques' into an artful and holistically comprehensive approach to the client's unique overall pattern. Chronic problems especially involve diverse tissues over wide areas of the body, and cannot be dealt with effectively solely by local treatment at the site of pain or dysfunction.

Developing the visual and palpatory assessment skills to create such bodywide session or series strategies with techniques such as these is the goal of our short courses and longer trainings (see Resources).

Introduction to the Fascial Webbing

Fascia is the missing element in the movement/stability equation. Understanding fascial plasticity and responsiveness is an important key to lasting and substantive therapeutic change.

Although anatomy books and technique libraries (including this one) are quick to label and identify these discrete bits, it is important to remember that humans are not constructed from parts like an automobile or computer. No 'part' of a biological creature could exist without constant and unbroken connection to the whole.

All One Net

Your fascial webwork began as a unified whole about the second week of your development, and will remain a single connected web from top to toe and from birth to death. From the moment of its inception, it has been folded and refolded in the complex origami of embryological development into a human who can stand, eat and read on its own. When we identify the different parts of this webbing – your dura mater, lumbar aponeurosis, mesentery, iliotibial tract or plantar fascia – we need to remember these are man-made names for subsets of your indivisible whole.

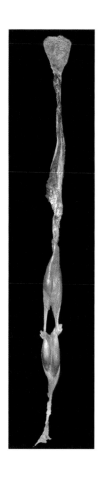

While every anatomy lists around six hundred separate muscles, it is more accurate to say that there is one muscle poured into six hundred pockets of the fascial webbing. The 'illusion' of separate muscles is created by the anatomist's scalpel, dividing tissues along the planes of fascia – and in the process obscuring the uniting element of the fascial webwork (figure 1.2). Of course these distinctions are useful, but this reductive process should not blind us to the reality of the unifying whole.

After birth, this single 'organ' is subject to the shadowless force of gravity – perhaps the largest force in shaping it, for better or for worse – interacting with the possibilities offered by our genes and the opportunities (or lack thereof) offered by our environment. It can be torn by injury or cut with a surgeon's blade, and it will do its best to self-repair. It shapes itself around our patterns of movement in breathing, walking, occupation and avocation. It is shaped by our psychological attitudes, by the movements they allow and do not allow. Finally, it is subject to the inevitable depredations of aging – degeneration, fraying and drying out – until we are finally ready to leave it behind.

Figure 1.2: The Superficial Back Line in dissection. Turn the scalpel on its side and you can readily see the fascial connections which link muscles in longitudinal series – part of the single net of fascia that runs from the toes (bottom) to the nose (top).

Through all of this it will remain a single, unifying and communicating network, holding us in a characteristically recognizable and physiologically viable shape, turning the contraction of the muscle tissue into sensible movement by transmitting it to the bones and joints, and in concert with the nerves and muscles generally managing the constantly changing mechanical forces that impinge on us via our contact with the rest of the world.

You cannot remove a cubic centimeter from the body's meat without bringing along some of this fascial net. This fascial system, which combines tough fibers with an amorphous gel of gluey proteoglycans (ground substance) in an aqueous medium, provides the environment for each and every cell, invests every tissue, surrounds every organ and binds the whole system into shape. With its intimate connection to every tissue structure, it also has a large role in physiological maintenance and immunity, but we will leave these roles for others to explain and focus on its mechanical functions.

Fascial Elements

To deal with this wide variety of forces, our connective tissue cells create an equally wide array of building materials by modifying a few surprisingly simple elements. Bone, cartilage, tendon, ligament, heart valves, sheets of tough fabric that surround the muscles, delicate gluey webbing that supports the brain, the transparent cornea of your eye and the dentin in your teeth – all of these and many other structures are made by connective tissue cells (figure 1.3).

Tissue type	Cell	Fiber types (insoluble fiber proteins)	Interfibrillar elements, ground substance, water-binding proteins
Bone	Osteocyte, osteoblast, osteoclast	Collagen	Replaced by mineral salts, calcium carbonate, calcium phosphate
Cartilage	Chondrocyte	Collagen and elastin	Chondroitin sulfate
Ligament	Fibroblast	Collagen (and elastin)	Minimal proteoglycans between fibers
Tendon	Fibroblast	Collagen	Minimal proteoglycans between fibers
Aponeuroses	Fibroblast	Collagen mat	Some proteoglycans
Fat	Adipose	Collagen	More proteoglycans
Loose areolar	Fibroblasts, white blood cells, adipose, mast	Collagen and elastin	Significant proteoglycans
Blood	Red and white blood cells	Fibrinogen	Plasma

Connective tissue cells create a stunning variety of building materials by altering a limited variety of fibers and interfibrillar elements. The table shows only the major types of structural connective tissues, from the most solid to the most fluid.

Figure 1.3: Cells such as fibroblasts and mast cells form connective tissues by altering the elements in the interstitial space, by altering the proportions of the constituent elements: fibers, gluey proteoglycans and water.

Using proteins supplied by our food via the bloodstream, connective tissue cells turn out the ubiquitous intercellular elements that hold our trillions of cells together. The principal element of our structure is tough collagen fiber, which is interwoven with other fibers – elastin and reticulin – in a bed of gluey mucopolysaccharides, also manufactured by these cells. These large sugar and protein polymers bind various amounts of water to create many configurations with a spectrum of properties that serve our varying needs for stability and mobility.

In bone, the leather-like dense web of collagen is embedded in an apatite of calcium and mineral salts that replaces the ground substance, producing the most rigid yet still resilient tissue in our bodies – the memento mori that lives on after us when our other tissues have melted away. Cartilage has the same leathery base (though cartilage can vary with more or less collagen, or elastin) but the rest of the interstitial space is filled with a silicon-like chondroitin.

In tendon and ligament, the fiber predominates, with only a small amount of glycoproteins within the network of fibers arranged in regular crystalline rows. In aponeuroses, there is a similar proportion of fiber to glycoproteins, but the fibers run every which way, like felt.

In the loose tissues, like areolar tissue or fat, fibers are interspersed within larger amounts of aqueous glycosaminoglycans. The lower viscosity in these tissues allows for easy dispersion of a variety of metabolites and infection-fighting white blood cells.

Within limits, the connective tissue system is able to modify these elements to deal with locally changing mechanical conditions, creating stronger ligaments and denser bones in response to the demands of (say) a summer dance camp, and of course to heal wounds, mend broken bones, or repair torn fabric. Unfortunately it can also modify itself in a downward direction as well, in response to a sedentary lifestyle, or a psychologically or occupationally based chronic pattern of holding.

Recently we have learnt that the cells themselves, at least a special brand of fibrocytes called *myofibroblasts*, can actually modify themselves to tie into the fascial webbing they have created via the integrins we discuss on page 13, and exert a force to contract it (figure 1.4). Up until this was discovered, it was assumed that muscle was contractile, but the fascia was passively plastic. Now we know that under certain conditions the fascia can contract, by means of these cells altering themselves to be like smooth muscle cells, and exert a contractile force into the surrounding fascial net.

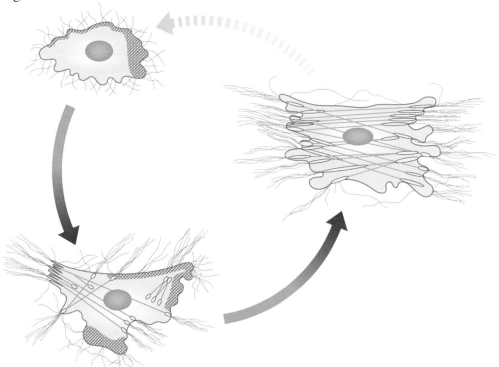

Figure 1.4: Myofibroblasts add cellular contraction to our picture of the fascial net. Under certain conditions, some fibroblasts hook their cellular structure into the connective tissue matrix, and then exert a slow, smooth muscle-like contraction into the fibrous webbing.

These conditions are very interesting, because unlike any other muscle cells in the body – smooth, cardiac, or skeletal – these hybrid connective tissue cells are not innervated. Instead of being stimulated by nerves, they are stimulated either by certain chemicals like antihistamines or oxytocin, or by sustained mechanical tension through the fascia they are connected into.

Myofibroblasts take some time to build into such a contraction – twenty minutes minimum – and some hours to completely let go, so this is not an immediate compensatory contraction such as we might see in other muscle tissue. But the combined contraction of many myofibroblasts does exert a significant pull on such large sheets as the crural fascia around the lower leg, the thoraco-lumbar fascia in the lower back, or the palmar or plantar fascia, where overactivity of these cells may contribute to fibromatosis or Dupuytrens' contracture.

While little is currently known about the clinical implications of the presence or contraction of myofibroblasts and what it might indicate for the manual therapist, it does represent a significant departure from the established ideas, and shows us that what we 'know' about the fascia – i.e. it does not actively contract – is subject to change.

Fascial Signaling

The biochemical signaling that governs such tissue changes on the cellular level is just yielding its secrets to researchers, but the implications of this new mechanobiology are far-ranging for all manual and movement therapists. Every cell, and especially every fibrocyte, is not only 'tasting' its surrounding chemical milieu (à la the work of Candace Pert et al. (1997) with neuro-peptides), it is 'listening' and responding to the mechanical environment of tensions and compressions as well.

The mechanism through which this happens is via special molecules that stud the surface of most cells in the body, but especially the fibroblasts and their cousins, called *integrins* (figure 1.4). Cells fix themselves within the connective tissue net via integrins. Cells move through the body primarily by reaching out to make new integrin connections at their 'head' end and loosening those connections at the 'tail' end. The integrins are connected via the cytoskeleton deep into the cell, such that new pulls of the connective tissues can affect the cell's behaviour, and even how its genes express themselves.

The implications of this finding are profound. It suggests that we could define structural health as a state where each cell of the body lives in its ideal mechanical environment. What constitutes 'ideal' varies from cell type to cell type, and can even vary within cell types in different parts of the body.

Muscle cells like a bit of tension in their environment; most nerves work best in low-tension situations. Epithelial cells will express their genes differently in a more tensional environment than they do in a more compressed one.

At the extremes, cells put under too much tension tend to abandon their 'job' in favor of reproducing more of themselves to resolve the high tension. Cells that are too compressed tend to commit suicide (apoptosis) in preference to forming a tumor, which is what happens when cells are too crowded.

The ancients searched for the proper proportion of the human body, looking at the golden mean and the relative proportions of different parts of the body. Now, we can define a new ideal of proportion based on the optimal biomechanical environment for each cell. While we are a long way from being able to measure this in a therapeutically specific way, this concept points to an exciting new marriage between cellular biology and manual therapy.

Another form of fascial signaling stems from the idea that the wet collagenous network forms a liquid crystal, a semi-conducting network. Pressure or tension creates an ionic flow within this web, known as *piezo-electricity,* and this electrical flow stimulates or depresses the fibroblasts to form (or not form) new fibers (figure 1.5).

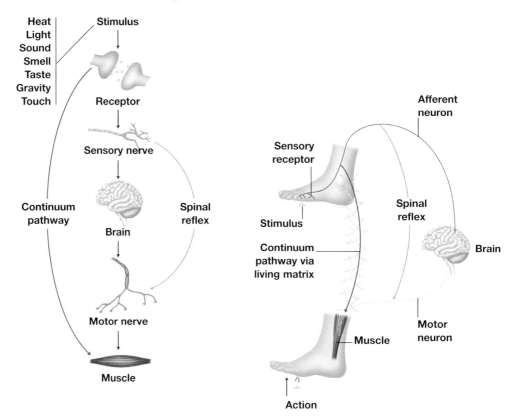

Figure 1.5: We have long acknowledged the neural net as a signaling network, but the connective tissue network is potentially a second, perhaps more primitive but five times speedier, signaling network.

In this way, the tension of our movements, especially oft-repeated movements, allows 'remodeling' of our connective tissues, including the bones and ligaments, when we put ourselves through the summer dance camp in our example above, or more subtly as our posture changes due to change of occupation, a psychological attitude, or advancing age.

Thus, when we enter the client's neuro-myofascial web, we are seeking to augment or steer natural processes in a direction helpful to healing or more efficient performance, from the cellular and molecular level all the way up to biomechanical whole of performance – daily, athletic or artistic.

In terms of the overall neurology – although the effect of deep touch on the many neural receptors in fascia (most of which are modifications of stretch receptors) has not been finally settled – the general effect seems to be to reset the 'tone-o-stat' of the nerves, restoring sensation in unresponsive nerves, and lowering the stimulation threshold of motor nerves that are stuck in the 'on' position (figure 1.6).

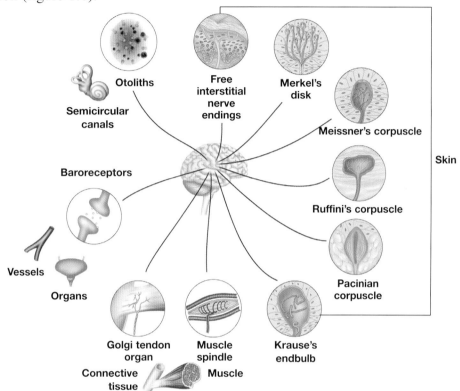

Figure 1.6: Your fascia is your richest sensory organ, filled with nerves including free nerve endings, Golgi tendon organs, Pacinian corpuscles, Krause's endbulbs, and Ruffini's corpuscles – all giving the brain a clear picture of the pressure, vibrations, shear – in fact, any deformation of the fascia.

In the fascia, the effect of deep touch seems to melt the glycoproteins that have become more viscous, and through their thixotropic quality, they can reverse back to a more malleable gel-like, less gluey viscosity. The connective tissue is a complicated colloid that could be compared to a gelatin dessert: put it in the fridge and it hardens; put it on the stove and it liquefies (becomes thixotropic). A similar process is happening in touch (and probably in dynamic exercise and yoga-like stretching as well).

When deep touch is applied with a specific directional vector, the melting of the glycoproteins between the fibers allows the collagen fibers to slide on each other, creating a plastic deformation that results in a sustained lengthening of the tissue. This is quite different – in intent, feel, and result – from stretching elastic muscle tissue. It is this plasticity in the fascia that accounts for the permanence and progressive nature of well-ordered fascial manipulation. Unlike muscle, fascia – once it is successfully lengthened – does not 'snap back' into place.

It requires a sustained touch to get the fascia to melt and move, and the specific depth and direction of tissue stretch is vital. Deep touch also affects the many nerve endings in the fascia, and the lengthening effect may proceed from the neurological effect or the thixotropic effect or some combination of both. This book is designed to guide you into a feel for the tissue changes and direction that will give you the maximum result for the minimum effort.

In summary, the nerves, muscles and fascia combine to make myofascial tissues a dynamic place to be. Deep touch can affect all three of these tissues, but the effect on the fascia, when melted and lengthened, is sustained, giving the other two tissues time to readjust to the new mechanical environment. Fascial tissue as a whole – cells, fibers and 'glue' – can be deformed by injury, abuse or disuse, but the good news is that it is 'plastic' – it can be reformed in response to skilled bodywork, stretching and awareness.

This section has gone some way in explaining the local effects of mechanical strain and therapeutic release on the connective tissues, where every cell, as we mentioned, is now known to be 'listening' and adjusting to the mechanical messages coming in from all around it. Additionally however, as therapists, we routinely see that work in one part of the body can cause shifts in some other part of the body quite distant from the site of applied manipulation. For example, work in the ankles may provide relief in the lower back, or opening in the neck may result in a more expanded breathing pattern.

To see how local changes can produce global results, we need to return to the idea of the fascia being all one net, and see the entire design in light of an unusual kind of engineering we use in our bodies called 'tensegrity'.

Tensegrity

The body is designed to distribute strain globally, not to focus it locally. The immediate forces of exertion in gravity, as well as the more slowly moving forces of compensation for injury and patterns of use, are best understood in terms of a particular type of geometry known as 'tensegrity'.

Dealing with tension, compression, bending and shear is the daily bread of engineers. Ever since Descartes, our body has often been described in terms of a 'soft machine', where the bones are like girders, the muscles like cables, and the whole structure somewhat like a crane – a series of pulleys and levers understandable in terms of Newton's laws of motion and (at a deeper level) thermodynamics. While this mechanical approach to kinesiology has given us much insight into the biomechanics of movement, such an analysis has not really clarified even such simple actions as walking. It certainly does not shed light on the kinds of global compensation for insult we are discussing here.

The advent of chaos mathematics, fractal equations, and greater understanding of how living systems hover on the edge of complexity has led to a new understanding of the human stability/mobility dynamic. Rather than seeing the body in the same terms as we see our houses and bridges, we can instead view the body as an example of a unique type of structuring known as '*tensegrity*' (a neologism derived from 'tension' and 'integrity'), in which the integrity of the structure rests on the balance of tensional forces, rather than a continuity of compressional forces.

Initiated by artist Kenneth Snelson, and developed by designer Buckminster Fuller, tensegrity structures give a contrasting way to see ourselves. Instead of viewing the skeleton as a sturdy framework (which it clearly is not – even the classroom skeleton has to be wired together and hung from a stand) from which the muscles hang, we can see the body as a single tensional webwork, in which the bony struts 'float' (figure 1.7).

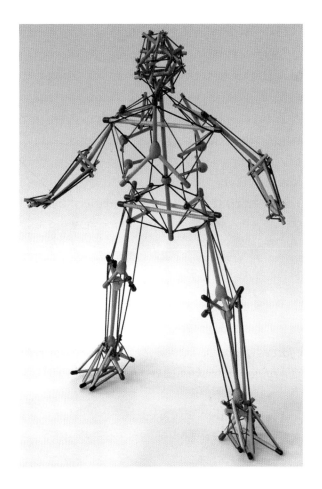

Figure 1.7: A new model of human structure – a tensegrity model in which the bones 'float' in a sea of soft tissue tension (model and photograph courtesy of Tom Flemons, www.intensiondesigns.com). This structure behaves like humans in some very interesting ways.

Verbal descriptions of tensegrity soon get tangled. Pictures help, but playing with, handling, or building a tensegrity structure is the best way to get a sense of how these structures work (figure 1.8).

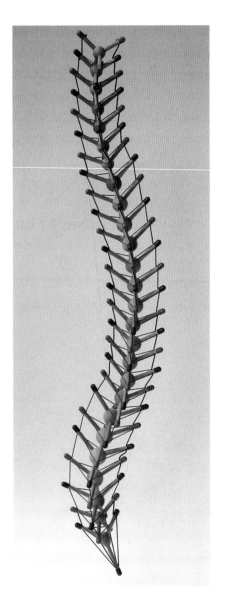

Such structures are more resilient than the cranes or machines we are usually compared to, and display several unique properties that recommend them as a model for human functioning:

1. Internal integrity

Your house or a crane would not work as well if it were turned upside down, but an animal body, including a human, maintains its structural integrity while hanging from a tree, doing a headstand, or spinning through a dancer's airy leap. Tensegrity structures, because of the internal balance of tension and compression, similarly hold their shape no matter what their orientation.

2. Strain distribution

Because the elastic bands in a tensegrity structure are continuous and the compression members ('bones') float in isolation, any deformation (caused either by pushing on a bone or changing the tension on a single string) will create strain that is distributed evenly throughout the structure. This results in small amounts of deformation over the whole structure rather than large amounts of deformation locally.

Figure 1.8: The spine modeled as a tensegrity structure. Obviously these simple models only begin to rival the complexity of the spine, but in action they mimic certain aspects of our own movement and behavior in both function and dysfunction.

This phenomenon has been demonstrated biologically (Huijing 2009), and in this writer's opinion is highly under-rated in current treatment texts. In short, any injury rapidly becomes a distributed phenomenon patterned into the whole body, and requires a whole-body assessment, and whole-body treatment. A whiplash is a problem of the neck for a few days, a problem of the spine for a few weeks, and thereafter a whole-body problem. Continuing to treat only the neck after this period is an all-too-common mistake.

3. Expansion or contraction in all axes

Squeeze a balloon around its center, and it becomes longer. Pull on a rope, and its girth decreases as the tension is increased. Because of their distributive quality, tensegrity structures act differently (and often, so do bodies). Expand a tensegrity structure in one dimension, and it will sometimes (depending on its internal structure) expand in all directions. Compress it, and it will compress not only along the line of force, but in all dimensions, becoming denser and more resilient as it does.

Bodies show this kind of phenomenon also. A body with a serious injury can contract and retract along all its axes, not just the one the insult first encountered. On the other hand, as we open the body in one dimension, it seems to expand into all dimensions – more height, more width, more depth.

Although the final verdict is not in on exactly how the body's mechanics work, seeing the body in terms of tensegrity leads to coherent global strategies that greatly enhance the efficacy and longevity of local treatment.

Though the fascia is very important in all the respects we have mentioned – its plasticity, its resilience, its communication and its holistic nature – it is not, of course, the entire picture. We can go some way toward filling in the 'fibrous body' by adding the two other whole-body systems, the circulatory and nervous systems. These two systems are more widely understood than the fascial system, and our muscles are clearly tied to the neural signals and nutritional bloodstream for their function. Thus, most locomotor therapies have concentrated on the free flow of fluids to and from the cells or the coordination of movement via unimpeded nerves (figure 1.9).

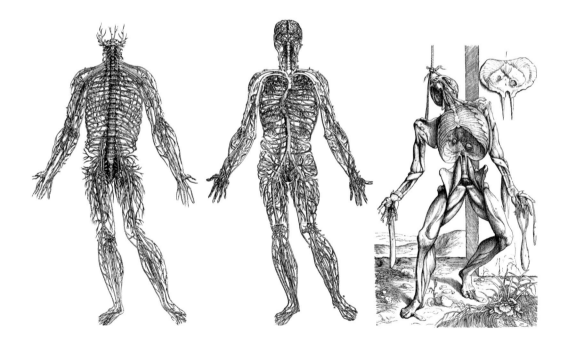

Figure 1.9: The three whole-body networks were outlined by Vesalius, who published slightly before this book in 1548. In his wonderful etchings, we see how any of these nets would show us the shape of the whole body. The fascial net is the least developed of these three images, and remains so over 450 years later.

Of course these well-documented effects on what is in fact a seamless neuro-myofascial web are very important, and in practice impossible to completely separate. Nevertheless, our thesis is based on the properties of the fascial part of this web that mediates between stability and mobility.

Compared with these other networks, the fascial network is at once faster to communicate – 720 mph for mechanical information versus 150 mph for the nervous system – but slower to respond than either the neural or vascular. The fascia's remodeling response is measured in days and weeks, rather than seconds or minutes. It is slow to accept changes initiated from the outside, and holds on to what changes it makes. This makes the fascial system a repository of much of the patterning for chronic issues, as opposed to the acute. Of course, there can be acute trauma to the connective tissues, as in a broken bone, severed tendon or sprained ligament, but the effect of this trauma distributes itself across the tissue webbing and tends to persist long after the initial healing of the other tissues.

The inflammatory response that both swells and brings healing proteins to damaged tissue also leads eventually to increased fibrosis, the loss of available movement between layers, and a 'stickiness' to the interstitial elements that impedes vascular and lymphatic flow. Chronic tension caused by inappropriate fascial shortness or laxity can lead to neuromuscular trigger points, and the reverse is equally true: chronic tension from anxiety or occupational misuse, disuse, abuse or overuse can lead to fascial thickening.

In conclusion, though many approaches are valuable in intervening in the neuro-myofascial web, there is a case for considering the fascial component of both short-term and long-term therapy for structural imbalance (figure 1.10).

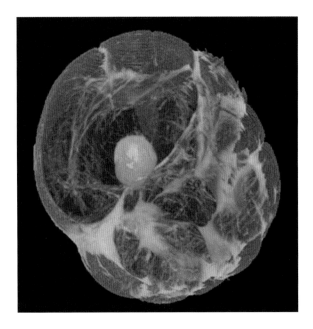

Figure 1.10: A modern rendition of the fascial net, done via computer by Jeff Linn using the Visible Human Data Project. Here we can see the thigh, a small section of what could be mapped in full: the fascial webbing of the body, which would include everything from the meninges through the organ bags and supports, the muscles' epimysia, endomysia and intermuscular septa, surrounded by the deep investing fascia and the superficial areolar and dermal layers.

Fascial Release and Developing Your Touch

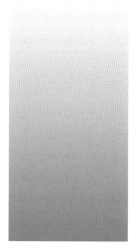

2

Touch is essential, a vital 'food' for the body and mind. It is needed to refresh us, steady us, comfort us and nurture us. Touch is required for most of our work and as a necessary method of communication as we make our way through the world. Much has been written of the many types of touch and much research carried out on its effects, but there is very little written on precisely how to develop safe, effective, and profound therapeutic touch to the fascial tissues.

This book is intended to be more than a listing of techniques; it is hopefully a catalogue of 'intentions', of ideas on how you can create different effects in the tissue by using alternate styles of touch. We will explore this more in the following section, but first we must look at how we touch, and begin to create a vocabulary to describe what it is that we do. There are many styles of touch: directive, informing, loving, nurturing, abusive, healing, calming, patronizing, or seductive. We can become richer therapists by developing our abilities to choose among a wide range of touch-abilities as possible.

Montagu (1986) in his classic text wrote about the nurturing effects of contact, well documented in the research literature and so well summarized by him, but very little has been written about the mechanics of our main method of therapeutic input. Different authors and teachers have emphasized various aspects of a stroke depending on their own experience. Chaitow (2006) talks of melting into the tissue; Hungerford (1999) warns us 'not to drop the connective tissue'; Myers (1999) talks about the three *I*'s of invitation, intention and information. But what is lacking is an adaptive model and vocabulary for all the elements in a complete stroke or intervention.

Our hope is that by using a staged model we can begin to put a language together that can facilitate discussion. With shared terms to express and explain the various methods we employ, we can, as individual practitioners and as a profession, become not only more conversant with the tissue and its wonderful variations, but also more conscious of the various stages we go through and the different types of information we give or receive in each stroke.

Under a skilled practitioner's hands, Fascial Release Technique (FRT) is a wonderfully releasing, pleasurable though occasionally challenging experience for the client. Like many tools, when wielded by a novice, it can be really quite uncomfortable. In order to avoid putting your clients through unnecessary discomfort, we recommend spending some time working through and playing with the five stages below. It is a common mistake to believe that the only thing that matters is 'getting the work done', but if we are to be a client-centered therapy, then surely it is our responsibility to stay aware of the fact that we are working on a person, not a collection of dysfunctional tissue crying out for our saving, healing and sometimes overeager touch.

The five-stage model is:

DASIE: Development, Assessment, Strategy, Intervention, Ending

This five-stage model may appear to be aimed at the novice practitioner. This is deliberate, in order that you can see where your style may differ or what you may be leaving out, and which aspects may be emphasized in your stroke to the detriment of others. We believe that even the most experienced practitioner can benefit from the analysis this model can bring.

This five-stage model was first developed as a counseling model (Nelson-Jones 1995); we have adapted it here for bodywork.

Stage 1. Development

Many bodywork approaches talk of 'melting' into the tissue and 'sinking through the layers', and FRT is no different. Be aware of the layers as you pass through them, allowing the tissue to give way rather than bulldozing your way through. Mold your hands, fingers, knuckles or whichever tool you are using to the shape of the body part being worked. Use only enough tension and pressure to reach that first layer of resistance, going slowly enough to be invited in.

In this stage you are developing your 'rapport' with the tissue. It is the initial engagement, the journey from being in the client's energetic field through each successive layer of tissue to get to the target structure. But it is also more than that; the process is mindful, sensitive to the transfer of energy (of whichever and any and all forms you are sensitive to), sensing that relationship and waiting for that invitation (Myers 2009) or the absorption into the sponge (an image used by Maupin [2005]).

Some schools teach that you can ask your client to exhale as you melt in, and we often find this a useful addition in difficult or challenging areas. If overused, however, the insistence on this element can be distracting rather than enhancing. Experiment using your own exhale to sink your bodyweight into the tissue. Having your center of gravity high and keeping your back heel raised will allow you to position yourself precisely over the desired area. Exhaling (quietly!) and dropping your center of gravity (or sinking your *hara*) is much easier for the client to receive than if you *muscle* into it with your arms and hands. The tension necessary to push will result in the client's tissue resisting, and sets up a struggle, however gentle, that one of you has to win.

Maintaining a relaxed point of contact avoids putting tension into the area being worked as it will try to resist you but also keeps you much more sensitive to variations in the myofascia. The less tone you have in your working limb, the better able you are to sense the changes in your clients.

Achieve this by getting as much of your force from muscles as distant from the point of contact as possible. For example, if you are using your fingertips they should retain only the tension needed to get through the layers. The initial force comes from your bodyweight coming over the area. As you need to reach deeper levels, increase your bodyweight by altering the angle of your back foot. Push from the ball of the back foot (remembering to engage your core), stabilize your shoulder girdle and arm, and gently lock your elbow and wrist. Only as a last resort should you push with your fingers, as that is more likely to feel 'pokey' and uncomfortable.

Stage 2. Assessment

So now that you have got 'somewhere' you need to check two things – first, is it where you wanted to be? If, for whatever reason, you were trying to find the fibularis muscles, how do you know that you are really on them? Second, if you are on them, how do they feel? What kind of work do they need, and what kind of tool should you be using? Would it be better to use your fingers, knuckles or elbow?

This is the stage of asking questions and obtaining information. Using both active and passive movement, you can gain much of the information you need. Asking your client to invert/evert the foot as you search for the fibularis muscles can help you differentiate them from the soleus. Feeling for the quality of the movement, you can assess which parts of the muscle open too much or not at all. You can begin to find the areas you will need to focus on, but how are you going to do it?

Pick (1999, cited in Chaitow & Fritz 2006) describes three tissue levels, surface, working and rejection, each of them being subsequently deeper than the next. They are not specific layers of the body but dependent on the level of dysfunction or sensitivity in any given area. The surface level mostly refers to the skin; the working level is where most bodywork interventions will take place; and the rejection level is when any resistance experienced is overridden or ignored by the practitioner and pain is experienced. The practitioner must decide at which of these levels they want or need to work. If it is within the rejection level, it should be negotiated with the client, preferably with the more superficial tissue addressed first to further prepare the area. Where these tissue levels exist can vary from area to area (depending on tissue condition), from day to day (depending on diet and stress level, and certainly from person to person (one person's surface is another person's rejection level). Stay sensitive in your assessment to identifying and knowing where you are relative to these levels.

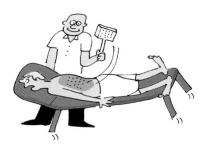

Figure 2.1: Sometimes it may be necessary to reach the 'rejection' layer, but it tends to be not as readily accepted by the client, particularly if it comes as a surprise.

Stage 3. Strategy

You are where you want to be with something that needs to be worked – but now you have to decide how you are going to do it. Which direction will have the best therapeutic effect? Which movement will you ask the client to make in order to help your stroke? Which tool (fingers, knuckles, forearm, etc.) will best fit the area? This is the stage of processing the gathered information into a coherent strategy.

Practitioners often skip the two stages of Assessment and Strategy; they are not discrete moments in time but merely part of a thought process, a mindful decision-making ensuring that your work is specific to the needs of the client rather than a treatment by rote. Of course, a certain amount of a 'recipe' is needed for beginning practitioners. Those of us from a massage background were given a basic sequence to get through the early days of practice, but as we became more comfortable with the techniques and more aware of their effects on the variations of individual clients and their tissue, we learnt to adapt that template to suit the presenting requirements. With FRT, this can and should be done with each and every stroke.

These are also stages that will become richer with experience. With each client and every venture into tissue, you are hopefully building your vocabulary of touch. Every time you strategise, stroke, and reassess, you have a palpatory experience of success or failure. You are laying down foundations of understanding which styles, strengths or other variations of touch will work (or fail) in each situation. If you ignore the strategy step, you can easily fall into habitual ways of working that eventually narrow your vocabulary and limit your touch-abilities. A pause to strategise helps to build a deep (and non-verbal) reference library – but the speed at which you create this reference tool will depend on how you proceed through the next stage, intervention.

Stage 4. Intervention

Finally, you reach the stage of doing the work. You are into and have checked the area you are working on, you have decided on how to work it, and now you can. As part of your strategy you have already chosen which tool to use. You are locked in the level and area you want to be, and now you slowly glide and/or ask the client to move. However, this stage is not so much about how you perform the stroke, but much more about what effect it is having. The practitioner has to constantly monitor what is happening below and around the point of contact. Is the tissue releasing? Is the right area being challenged with the movement? Is the tissue lifting or moving? Is the client able to receive and process the information you offer to her?

Throughout the intervention, or stroke, you set up a feedback loop assessing its effectiveness. What changes can you make as you go through to assist you in the goals set above? With each change you have to re-evaluate.

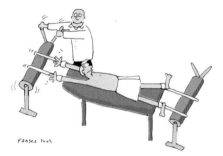

Figure 2.2: With each increase of intensity, the practitioner should be feeling for a little feedback.

Now you are truly listening to the client and their tissue, setting up what we sometimes refer to as a 'communication between two intelligent systems'. With your strategy in mind, you are offering information to the client, asking their tissue if it can change, and asking if the work makes sense to them. By listening to the collection of systems under your hand and keeping yourself open to their messages, you will be able to accommodate the abilities of the client's tissue in your work, providing you can attune your ear to the language their tissue uses to inform you in response to your contact.

Schwind (2006) encourages us to use as many of the other, non-working, surfaces of the hands as possible to aid this communication. Using the supporting hand as a *mother hand*, for a nurturing contact, or as a *listening hand,* is common among many bodywork traditions, but it is only of maximum benefit if it enters into part of this conversation. It should not be there just to provide comfort and ease, but to put the third dimension into what can otherwise be a two-dimensional stroke. Two hands working in coordination with a client's movement produce many times the therapeutic power of simply 'doing a stroke' with one hand.

This is how to grow the vocabulary of your touch, experimenting with all of the many variables and listening for the changes that take place. Schleip (2003) has shown us the many types of mechanoreceptors in the fascial tissue, and each will respond to different forms of stress in its surrounding fibers. We therefore need to learn how to talk to each of them, as they will have different languages.

Variation occurs among clients, and even within different areas of the same client. There will be variations in the type of dysfunction, as well as in the fascial layers or structures, whether regular or irregular, dense or loose, bound or hypermobile. Each has a different language (or dialect, at least), so the wider your vocabulary of touch, the clearer our conversation will be.

Stage 5. Ending

As you begin, so should you finish. If you take all that time to take care of your client, sinking in, feeling the tissue's condition and listening to it change as you work, then honor both the client and the work by coming out slowly. Sometimes it seems as though therapists forget that they are working with another person; sometimes it seems they are so relieved to reach the end of their stroke that they jump out of the tissue. We are not saying it is wrong, perhaps just a little sudden and impolite to the client. Take your bodyweight back into your forward leg; do not push into the client to jerk yourself up. Once you have your weight back in your legs then you can lift yourself out of the stroke, allowing the tissue time to settle in rather than letting it snap back.

Sometimes it can be more pleasant for the client to spiral (Aston 2006) out of the contact, slowly peeling your skin out of contact with theirs. This is especially true when you work in areas where the skin may be more sensitive, such as around the armpit or the thigh adductors.

This is just one style; remember that the exit is part of your intent. Even shocking the tissue could get the desired response, by either allowing a recoil effect or perhaps by increasing tone and awareness in the area. The important point is that it is a conscious decision and is coherent with your intention to create change with the client.

It is these small details that the client may not be aware of but that make a huge difference in their experience of the treatment. Fascial release can be a challenging treatment, and the more comfortable we can make it for the client, the better they will be able to accept it and embrace its benefits.

We fully realize that the model may seem formulaic for many intuitively driven practitioners; this is deliberate. We have to start being explicit about what it is that mysteriously draws us to the 'right' layer, informs us of which direction to work and with which tool. With mindful practice, we can build the 'intuition' that comes of unconscious competence, that heightened sensitivity that responds to the needs of the tissue through an innate sympathy with it. Our minds will gradually become attuned to the language of the tissue and rapidly go through these stages with very little conscious awareness on our part.

DASIE is not a technique, nor even a style of touch, but rather a way of describing the process as we interact with our clients' tissue. By doing so, we hope that we can bring even more depth to the three-dimensionality of our work. We aim to listen to the tissue at every stage and adopt, initially, a conscious direction to our work. As our expertise grows, we allow this to become a preconscious process, but never an unconscious treatment by rote. We should always be aware of the entire person and their many levels as we treat, being responsive to the needs of each level and reacting in such a way as to develop a three-dimensional communication through touch.

Fascial Release Technique

Having focused on how we enter and exit, we now need to look at the mechanics of FRT, because the style and intention of it differs from that of many other forms of bodywork. Generally when performing massage techniques, the therapist glides over the top of the myofascia, applying compression to the tissue in order to stimulate the flow of fluids and to affect neuromuscular tension (figure 2.3).

In order to manually stretch the connective tissue, the therapist needs to use a different style of contact. This is done by first applying a downward pressure, sinking to the first level that gives resistance and then dropping the angle of contact in order to create a wave in front of the point of contact (figure 2.4). This wave is then maintained in front as the stroke is performed. The stroke must be carried out slowly and at a speed determined by the interaction of the tool being used (thumb, forearm, elbow, etc.), the amount of lubrication available along the surface, and the rate at which the client's tissue can melt and open up as you work along.

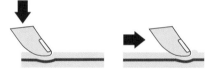

Figure 2.3: Massage stroke applying compression.

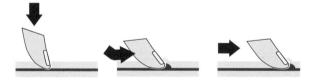

Figure 2.4: Fascial release stroke.

We sometimes think of it as taking an elevator down to the floor (tissue level) you want to be at. As you walk out the door, you drop the angle of contact, locking yourself into the myofascial layer and then continuing the conversation we discussed earlier between you and your client's tissue by performing the stroke.

We recommend experimenting with different types of lubricant, starting with only the moisture of your own hands. With too little lubrication, you will jerk or 'skitter' over the tissues and be unable to perform the stroke smoothly. If so, wet your hands with a little water. Only if this fails should you try a little moisturiser or wax-based lubricant (see Resources). Too much lubricant, and oil-based lotions or oils in particular, reduce your ability to grip the tissue, making FRT work difficult, painful and ineffective. Remember, always start with less, as it is easier to add a little more than to take it off if you use too much.

Fascial Layers

The client may feel a slow pulling and burning sensation – this is partly what you are trying to achieve as you 'melt' the ground substance within the myofascia to a more liquid state (changing it from 'gel' to 'sol') and stretch the connective tissue bag surrounding and within the target areas.

If you are unfamiliar with palpating the fascial coverings around the muscles, try exploring through the layers of your forearm. Using the fingers of your dominant hand, begin by first placing your awareness on the surface of the skin. Feel its resistance to your pressure, the tautness of the skin giving a positive sensation in response to the slight weight of your fingertips. Try moving the skin over the underlying adipose. Is it separate from the layer beneath? Does the skin move more easily in one direction than the other?

Now sink into the adipose layer. Become aware of the different quality of the sensations in your fingertips. How does this layer differ from being 'in the skin'? Press a little more firmly and you can feel another tight layer below this, more taut and bouncier than the skin. Can you move the adipose over this second skin? Feel how the skin and the adipose move easily together, gliding over this first layer of myofascia: the deep investing layer. Maintaining the pressure to keep your digits in the adipose tissue, angle your pressure toward your elbow, taking up any slack, and then slowly flex your wrist. Can you feel the stretch on the skin? With a firmer grip and more movement, you can feel how this type of contact can become uncomfortable. It is similar to an 'Indian' (or, in the UK, a 'Chinese') burn, so beloved of school playground bullies and older brothers the world over.

Once you recover from the slight abuse you have just given yourself (and hopefully not elicited too many traumatic memories!) allow your fingertips to descend through the layers again, this time overcoming the resistance given by the deep investing layer of fascia. You will feel yourself now pushing onto the muscle belly, using the tone of the muscle as your guide to assess which level you are on; the focus is the 'skin' of that first muscle you encounter. You can check to see if you are in the right layer by flexing your wrist again. Do you feel the muscles stretching below your point of contact similar to your first attempt, or do you feel the tissue around the fingertips pull them toward the wrist?

If you are in the correct layer, you can now begin applying FRT on your wrist extensors by 'hooking' the tissue, pushing toward your elbow as you slowly flex your wrist again. Be aware of the different sensations in the tissues between the two different levels of connection. If you have got it right, it should now feel like a deeper burning, but more pleasant. Sometimes clients report it as a 'good pain', the tissue almost crying out for the release, stimulation and stretch you are giving it.

To put it into the context of the DASIE model (page 22), you have melted into the tissue (Development), felt the appropriate layer (Assessment), decided which direction to lock and which movement to make (Strategy), and then done the work (Intervention), finally melting back out of the tissue to finish (Ending).

For each of the techniques in this manual, you should progress through the same process; all of them are mindful, nurturing and listening. With each intervention, you should be working at an appropriate level and having that same conversation, listening for the feedback loop and adjusting accordingly. Experiment on yourself to feel where you are on the surface level (too superficial to feel effective), and the rejection level (ow! get out), and in the working level (just right), a bit of a pleasant challenge. Please, while we will not repeat this in each description, never forget that you are in a constant relationship not just with the client but even more directly with their tissue, and both deserve to be heard. Each movement should be carried out with the same care and attention as that of the sculptor's chisel on irreparable marble.

You can now explore through all of the musculature of the forearm. Feel for the differences in tone, not just in the muscle but also that fascial skin, the epimysium. Compare the flexor compartment to the extensors. Use movement to find the intermuscular septum between the muscles. Use movement to identify exactly where you are playing with flexion and extension in combination with radial and ulnar deviation. What difference does it make in the tension produced under your working hand? Can you sense that certain directions of movement give a better challenge to the tissue? As you become more proficient in using the technique, through regular practice, all of this will give you information about the area you are working on, its condition and where you need to focus your attention. You will be able to subtly alter the angles of movement to make your work even more effective.

Body Mechanics

As we saw earlier, there are many different types of fascia: dense connective tissue, both regular and irregular, adipose and areolar. We will be working with them in their different manifestations within the body. Each of them having various qualities and abilities to change, they will respond to stress in unique ways, creating diverse symptoms within the tissues and through the rest of the body. It should be obvious, therefore, that not all fascia will be treated in the same way. We need to alter the type and style of contact to suit the nature of the tissue we are working with and to achieve different results.

For example, we can lift and drop planes of fascia (dense irregular) as if we were redraping the fascial fabric over the skeleton; we can divide septa that have become glued together (by the intermediate areolar tissue); and we can release the knots and nodules (adhered dense regular tissue within the myofascia) – all the ubiquitous signs of the trials and tribulations of life. Each of these will require a variation on the basic technique, by varying the angle or the amount of surface contact or the nature of the pressure used.

There are so many permutations and combinations for varying circumstance that it is impossible to display all of them here, and for that reason we recommend attending a full course to gain further mastery. It is also with this in mind that we present these ideas in this book. It is intended as an aide-mémoire for those who have attended such a workshop, and perhaps a pointer for a slightly different direction for some who are already accomplished in such an approach. For the novice practitioner, however, direct, hands-on guidance in this style is often necessary to have confidence in the basic skills on which these techniques are built.

Within this text it is our intention to give you an understanding not only of the mechanics of a technique but also of the clinical and structural reasoning for its application – the ability to go from the assessment phase to forming your strategy, as well as the tools to perform the intervention. The reader must, however, understand the obvious limitations of a book of this size; it cannot cover all eventualities. The ideas here act as templates to give you a framework for achieving a desired goal. Many of the illustrated directions of the strokes are perhaps the most commonly used, but they could quite easily be reversed or otherwise modified for a less common pattern. In other words, these are guidelines, not commandments written in stone.

The more that you understand of the nature of the variations of fascia, the better able you will be to adapt your contact to suit your desired goal. The aponeuroses, the deep investing layer, the large sheaths of tissue of the epimysium can be moved medially or laterally, lifted or dropped, and they can be separated from the underlying tissues, but they will predominantly require a flatter, broad-surface contact, such as the heel of the hand or the ulnar blade. The lengthening of bound or adhered myofascia calls for a more precise point of contact. Fingers, or knuckles, are ideal for applying a focused release or following a tight line of tissue, and often a more assertive approach is used. The encouragement of the areolar tissue to open and divide within an intermuscular septum can require a coaxing, teasing, insinuating touch, using a tool slender enough to weasel its way between the adhered structures.

To get a picture of this, imagine how you would deal with a crooked tablecloth. When adjusting its position on the table, you would use both hands spread out to give a broad contact. But if it had not been washed since the last time you had a party for the kids, it might have a few folds and creases in it that had stuck together because of anonymous spilt substances. In this case, you would use a more precise contact to unknit the adhered surfaces. Engage the client with your weight more than your strength. In a way FRT is a 'lazier' form of bodywork, because both your sensitivity and the client's sensation depend on using a minimum of effort in your strokes. Having ease in your body-use is one of the essential elements for making the work pleasant to receive, and for prolonging your ability to do it and thereby extending your career span. The more you allow gravity to do the work, the less tension you will have to put into your point of contact. This will also make you more sensitive to changes in your client's tissue and give the client a softer contact.

One important aspect of this is the use of your back leg. It should be more or less straight, and your heel should be raised a little. Many schools seem to teach a flat-footed approach, as it is more stable to push from. But our experience shows that by lifting your pelvis – and, therefore, your center of gravity – you will need to 'push' less, and can achieve the movement by simply relaxing your forward leg to allow your bodyweight and gravity to do the work for you. You can then adjust your height by lifting or lowering your back heel, either giving more reach or dropping the angle of contact, and you will have the further advantage of allowing the spine to remain straight rather than hinging on a longer stroke.

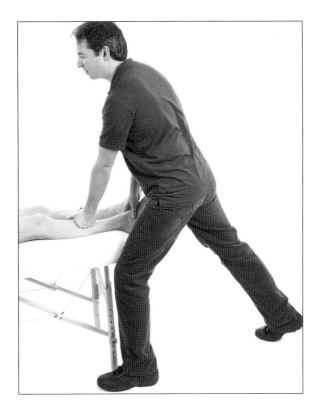 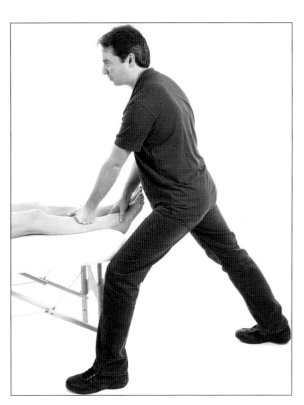

Figure 2.5a & b: a) Note how the back foot is raised to allow the body to be up, over the point of contact, allowing the body to sink in; b) the heel is then lowered to create the forward angle for the stroke, locking the contact at the correct layer.

As we discussed earlier, getting hooked in at your point of contact is necessary to lock you into the tissue. You can accomplish this easily by having your heel high as you sink into the tissue and then dropping it slightly to lower your angle and get the wave in front of your hand, elbow or forearm.

After you have engaged the tissue, then all of your upper body gently stablizes to maintain correct form, but it should do this in what seems like the reverse of your natural instinct. Many novice therapists want to push on the tissue as firmly as possible, and therefore lock their hands and give a hard feel to the client. But if you can relax your hands as much as possible and work initially from your waist and the center of gravity in your pelvis, or your *hara*, then you can maintain a soft contact, with the force coming from as far away from the client as possible. Your thighs, particularly the front one, will be controlling much of the weight.

Not only does this feel much more comfortable for the client but it also opens you to being much more sensitive to the client's tissue and any responses they may make as a result of your work. Because the existing tension on your muscle spindles affects their responsiveness to changes in tension, the less tension you have at your point of contact, the more receptive, and therefore responsive, to subtle changes you will be.

Use of the Hand

A full hand or the heel of the hand can be a very useful tool to work with the large expanses of fascial sheets. The broad contact allows an encompassing grip.

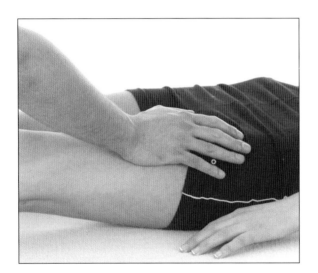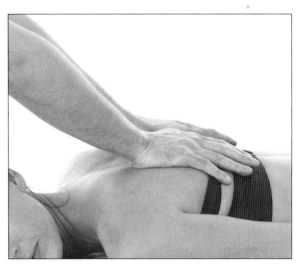

Figure 2.6a & b: a) The hands and the heels of the hand in particular are useful for moving the superficial sheets of fascia and for warming and preparing the tissue prior to more specific and deeper work, b) the angle at the wrists should be kept quite low to minimize strain on the joint and surrounding tissue, allowing the force to be transferred through the carpals from the forearm.

Use of the Fingers

Your fingers are neurologically the most sensitive tool you have, but mechanically the most easily abused. It is very important that you keep your fingers in neutral or slightly flexed. Never allow them to go into extension, as you will challenge their ligamentous integrity and eventually the joints themselves. (This hyperextension may happen inevitably at first, but please work toward the slight flexion as soon as you can.) In figure 2.7, note how the wrist is also kept in neutral. All of the force of the movement is transferred in a straight line from your elbows, through the bones of the carpals and metacarpals, into the phalanges. Adjustments in angle come from your shoulders by way of lifting or dropping your back foot.

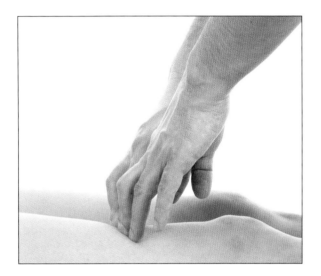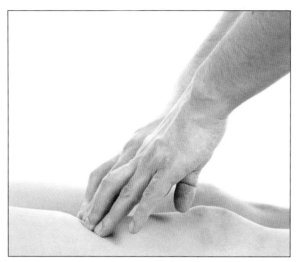

Figure 2.7a & b: Note not only the change in angle to engage the tissue from (a) to (b), but also how the hands and fingers remain slightly flexed or extended. Never hyperextend any of the joints.

The first few times you perform this type of stroke, you may feel the skin being pulled from under your nails. This eases with practice, and may be a sign that you are working too hard or need a little water or wax to help with the stroke, as the skin may be slightly dry and giving too much resistance. With practice, you learn many of the subtle alterations that can be made to minimize this.

Use of the Fist

Your fist is often overlooked or undervalued as a tool, and when it is used, it often carries too much tension and loses a lot of its potential sensitivity.

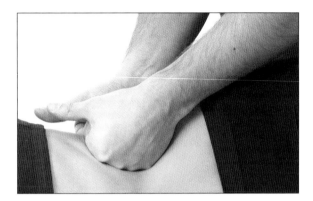

Figure 2.8: Even over the relatively thin tissue of the lateral thorax and working over the sensitive ribs, a relaxed fist can be a very useful tool. The hand should be brought to the body with little if any tension in it, the fingers open, not held in the fist. The client's body then shapes the practitioner's contact, rather than the other way around.

Once again the wrist joint is held in neutral, but this time changes in the angle can be achieved by using a scooping motion from the shoulder and by flexing the elbow as well as changing the height of the shoulders.

The fingers making the fist are held softly outside the palm, not folding inside as you would if forming a punch. This gives the fist the softness to mold to the shape of the client, allowing their tissue to push your fingers away, rather than holding your fingers in flexion and using more muscle tension than necessary in your forearm and hand.

When using the fist it is important to keep your thumb facing forward. The common mistake is to use the fist with the knuckles forward, but this puts a lot of strain into the wrist extensors. The pressure, weight or force is focused on the proximal aspect of the proximal phalange, close to the metacarpophalangeal joint of the index and middle fingers. Occasionally with raking types of strokes, when the practitioner's body goes over the point of contact (such as with the back stripes, page 202), then the palm will be facing forward.

Use of the Elbow and Forearm

The forearm is a great tool for large areas such as the back and the thighs, where sheets of connective tissue and large muscle groups can be moved and released.

You can adjust the focus of the point of contact on rounded areas like the thigh by flexing or extending your elbow to rock across the area – similar to changing the bowing on a violin (figure 2.9a & b). For more specific areas of restriction, precision and an easy sense of power can be achieved by using whichever surface around the point of the elbow makes a comfortable and fitting contact with the tissue you want to reach (figure 2.9a).

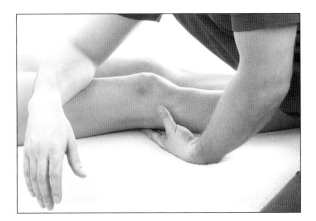 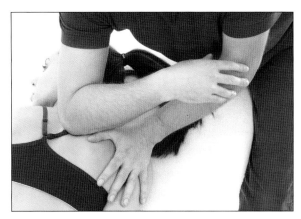

Figure 2.9a & b: Using the forearm and elbow. In (a), notice how the aspect of the quadriceps being addressed could alter by simply lifting or dropping the right wrist to change the angle of the forearm.

In contrast, figure 2.9b shows the use of the point of the elbow. Both photographs illustrate the different uses for the non-working hand, to guide the client's movement (figure 2.9a) and/or to guide the point of the elbow, ensuring accuracy and stability (figure 2.9b). In both cases the contact of the non-working hand can assist in comforting the client, but it also acts as another receiver for information regarding the client's experience, by listening for any protective flinches or tuning into the ease of the surrounding tissues.

For this technique it is important to keep your shoulders behind the stroke, sinking into it rather than dragging it through the tissues with your shoulder muscles.

Use of the Knuckles

While the elbow may be the strongest tool available for your use, it can often be relatively blunt in comparison to the knuckles of the index and middle fingers. To maintain their strength and stability, the knuckles are best used with an internal rotation of the humerus and pronation of the radio-ulnar joint to bring the little finger into the leading position (rather than the thumb, as when using the fist). This will give support to these two digits, allowing the bones of the proximal phalanges of the index and middle fingers, wrist, radius and ulna (and in most cases the humerus as well) to all be aligned. This provides maximum bony support, taking stress off the soft tissue and allowing the muscles to be relaxed for maximum sensitivity. For short strokes or stuck spots, your knuckles are tools of great versatility which can be used in a variety of positions.

As with the use of the fist, the distal phalanges which are not being used are pushed back by the client's tissue, not held back in flexion by the therapist.

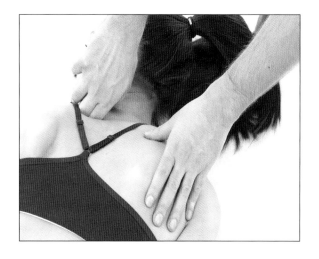

Figure 2.10: Note how the joints are all aligned from the elbow to the middle knuckles (proximal interphalangeal joints). The end of the stroke is reached at the point at which any of these joints need to bend to reach the target tissue. Reposition yourself to maintain correct body mechanics rather than sacrifice your own body.

Questions of Direction

There are many views on what can be done with FRT. We will sometimes refer to lifting or dropping tissue and moving it medially or laterally. We will release tissue, lengthen it in various ways, and spread it in others.

In many situations we want to change the relationship within the deep investing layer, that body stocking just below the skin and adipose layers. These planes of tissue require quite a different style of touch compared to when we wish to release the more specific tissue within a myofascial unit (a more accurate, if cumbersome, description than the common term 'muscle').

To move the large sheets of fascia, we need to use a larger, often softer, contact, and imagine taking hold of a skin under the actual skin. We sink to its level and lift or move the whole of that area. This can be done with the deep investing layer and sometimes with the epimysium of the muscles, but rarely within the muscles themselves. It is a sculpting, reshaping intention that you want to portray with your hands. Encourage the tissue to alter – sometimes it is nurturing, sometimes encouraging – almost as if you were remolding the body from modeling clay.

These types of strokes are not included within the main body of the text as they are quite specific to the shape of the client, and this is part of the artistry of the work. An outline for the use of the hands is given above. We encourage you to explore the use of this type of contact in different areas of the body, as it is a useful adjunct to and preparation for the more specific techniques that are discussed in the rest of this book.

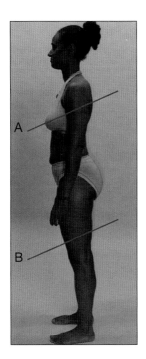

In figure 2.11, a comparison of the planes of fascia shows that the levels are lower in the front than the back in both the thigh and over the sternum. If you were to take a cross section through these areas and keep it at the same anatomical level (lines A & B) then you would have to angle the section downward to match the anterior tilt of the femur. This is quite different from the work that we would need to do with the flexors of her hip in correcting the anterior tilt of her pelvis. They require lengthening, and we could work to release them by engaging the tissue in both directions.

Figure 2.11: A side view of a client showing differences in the relationship of the deep investing layer between the front and back of her body.

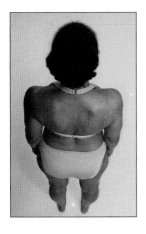

Figure 2.12: This superior view of the same model shows, among other issues, the medial rotation and anterior tilt of the shoulder girdles.

Our strategy to help ease the outer tissues of our model in figure 2.12 may include lifting the deep investing tissue up and out, as if we were re-placing the shoulders back to where they belong. This will then reveal the deeper issues held in the pectoralis major and pectoralis minor.

So we might start with the planar movement, using a broad finger or hand contact for the more superficial tissue remodeling (figure 2.13a & b) – but then if we need to address the deeper myofascia of the pectoralis major, we will want to use a slightly sharper or more specific tool (figure 2.13c & d). The fingers are still used in this example, but you can see the change in angle to sink more deeply into the pectoralis tissue.

You can see in figure 2.13c that the tissue is being stretched laterally as the arm is abducted. This is what we refer to as *assisting* the stretch. Both the movement of the tissue and the force of the engagement are going in the same direction. This will isolate the stretch in the tissue between your contact and the proximal attachment. If we make this into a stroke and glide laterally, then some effectiveness may be lost as the force of the stretch on the fascia is absorbed by an ever-increasing amount of this elastic tissue as you travel laterally away from the attachment.

If we reverse the engagement, aiming our intention medially (figure 2.13d) and resisting the active client stretch, this focuses the release in the tissue between our contact and the humeral, lateral attachments.

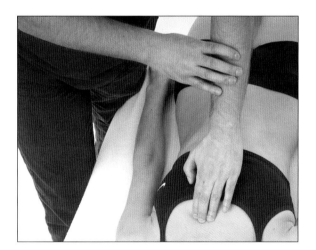
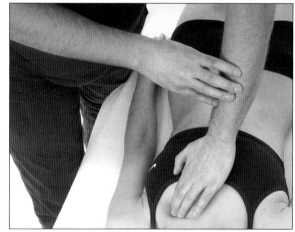
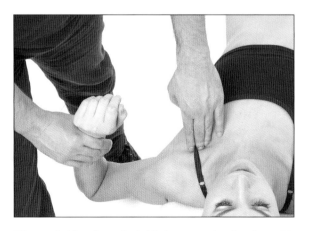
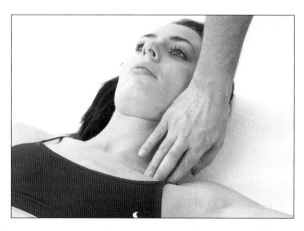

Figure 2.13a, b, c & d: Various methods of working the pectoral fascia in a range of directions with different tools.

Quite often we will need to differentiate tissue. Each layer within the body should be able to glide on another independently, but this ability can be lost for many reasons. Trauma, misuse or overuse, for example, can all lead to adhesions forming and restricting the adaptive nature of the adjoining areolar tissue. When this happens the body can have a 'locked' feeling in the area, and this is one of the reasons to use as much movement with the client as possible as you work. In certain areas we can spread the tissue to re-open septa (see adductor spreading, page 146), we can sink into the gap between structures to encourage release of any restrictions (see hamstring separation, page 106), or we can lock into one area and have the client move the underlying tissue to create a 'flossing' effect to gain release of the connective tissue and regain a smooth, differentiated relationship (see clearing the ankle retinaculum, page 69).

As discussed above, our touch will change depending on our intention and the nature of the tissue we are working with. The way we work with the dense regular tissue of the Achilles tendon will be very different from the teasing, swimming nature of sinking into the septa, and even this will differ among different septa of varying densities.

The competent therapist will be able to read not just the nature of the tissue but also the character of the client and what touch will produce the desired response. Constant attention and instantaneous adjustment of your touch are essential elements of good Fascial Release Therapy – assertive when required, nurturing when possible.

Designing a Session

A session should have a beginning, middle and end. A natural progression through the treatment helps put the client at ease and, as we will see, allows the preparation for and then integration of the main work contained within it.

Earlier in this chapter we looked at the DASIE model in terms of performing a single stroke, but we can also use it as a template for a session. The therapist initially **Develops** a relationship and rapport (or reconnects with a repeat client), then performs some form of **Assessment** by taking a case history, finding out what has happened since the last session, or in the case of fascial release work, performing a BodyReading visual postural assessment. This information is then used to develop the **Strategy** or treatment plan, which goals the therapist wishes to achieve in the session. Within the **Intervention** phase we experiment to see if it all matches and if we can achieve some of the desired goals, before bringing the session to an **Ending** with some settling treatment, such as neck, back or sacral work.

There can be many reasons for a client coming to see us, and the techniques contained within this book are not always suitable for working with acutely injured tissue. The reasoning behind our paradigm for working toward structural balance is that when we aid better alignment throughout the body, the tissue is less likely to be strained. The work is ideal for those with chronic musculoskeletal pain. Some clients can easily see the rationale for this, particularly if you use the mirror during the BodyReading as described below, but others may require more persuasion to see the logic of working somewhere completely different from where they experience pain.

At the outset, clarifying the goals of the client can help, as you can negotiate what is achievable and what may be expected from the treatments. Asking the client what their structural issues are and how they experience them, and finding a measurable and attainable goal for you both to work toward, can help both of you to focus on the session. Remember that you can have your client get on and off the table at any time (and hopefully more than once) during the session, in order to allow them to experience the work, to feel the differences, and for you to reassess the progress being made.

The Arc of a Session

The session usually progresses in an arc: from a sensitive beginning it gradually builds in intensity, the touch accessing ever deeper layers or more challenging areas before easing back to smoothing and integrating work at the end. It can be shocking to a client for the first contact to be in their psoas or their pectineus. Start with areas or structures that are more superficial and less intimate. Prepare the areas that need support. Prepare the client psychologically by beginning on areas that are more accessible or open to being touched – for most people, these will be the limbs or the back. You might know that you want to work with the pectoralis minor or the deep lateral rotators and they might be very familiar to you, but the chances are that the client will not be prepared for you to go straight there. Respect the arc, even with a familiar client; start easily and superficially, working up to the middle, more intense part of the session.

End Game

Always try to make sure you have some time left in the session after the most intense section to allow the client the chance to settle back into their body and integrate some of the changes that have taken place. As we mentioned above, this 'end game' normally consists of neck and/or back work, the pelvic lift, back stripes and occipital release in particular. The pelvic lift and occipital release are both relaxing and settling (and generally parasympathetically stimulating), and can of course be used in conjunction with the structural goals of the session; they are more than just nice strokes. The seated back work is a little more sympathetically stimulating, as the client has to support herself and be more actively engaged. The choice of which of these to use and in what order can be determined by the effect you wish or need to achieve for your client. If their system was aroused and they need to be more calmed, then focus on the neck and pelvic work; if they were seeming a little groggy and they need to drive after the session, then help bring them round with the seated back work, for example.

It is important that the client feels complete at the end of the session, and you contribute to this with how you progress through the session, as well as your choice of finishing strokes. Each session should be designed to work toward two or three goals – do not take on every structural issue in one session; do not jump all over the body from one limb to another, from the upper to the lower body and back again. Keep your work consistent. Work with one layer or one area and then have the client stand and feel the work. Then go deeper or balance it with work on the other limb, and repeat this process. Do not be afraid to talk with your client and have them move on and off the table. Our aim is to help them reconnect with their body, not disassociate from it.

After the session have your client walk or do familiar movements. Encourage them to tune into their body, and listen to any feedback they have. Reassess your goals: were they attained or not, and if not why not? How could the client support the work in the meantime? Are there habits that could be altered, e.g. seating positions in work or at home? What movements or stretches or awareness exercises could they be doing between now and the next session? Build a referral network of movement and exercise coaches, other bodyworkers to whom you can refer. In referring, pay careful attention to the needs and interests of the client. Not everyone wants to go to Pilates or yoga classes. Make sure, in assigning 'homework' that the path suggested is one with which the client will actually follow through.

Number of Treatments

We have all seen the Frankenstein-like pictures of those who have become addicted to plastic surgery. While we hope that our work would not produce results anything like that, take it as a warning for those that might get tempted to 'have just one more'. Many clients (and therapists) want to go ever further, to attain the perfect this or that. It is tempting to go along when the client appeals to your ego, when you see your dwindling bank balance or gaps in your diary. We strongly believe that there should be a beginning, middle and an end – an arc – to your series of sessions of structural work, and to your whole encounter with the client. It has to finish at some point, so it is best to approach this process consciously. Within structural integration that has been traditionally ten or twelve sessions, but it can be as few as three and sometimes just one.

The tools in this book are not designed to be used endlessly with the same clients. Many of the changes that can be created with them can take time to mature. Trust that they will, and encourage your client to do the same. Warning signs that you are doing too much of this kind of work with any given client include (1) all your sessions with them are beginning to look much the same – same areas, same strokes, same issues, or (2) you are getting diminishing returns from your sessions – it is just not as dramatic as it was in the beginning. Either of these should turn your attention to finishing this series with the client, and let them absorb your work for six months to a year, before you start again.

If you wanted a format for a simple three-session series, you might work (1) to balance the pelvis and lower limbs, then (2) to balance the rib cage and upper limbs, and finally (3) to balance the spine.

Single, one-off sessions can be very useful in supporting other work for acute problems. By bringing more symmetry to the area you can help take some of the accessory strain off. Beware, however, of removing compensation patterns that may be serving the client. These can be too complex and various to explain here, but working in cohort with any other practitioners involved in the client's care will help clarify your goals.

To learn the complexities of a full structural integration series, we recommend that you attend a full training (e.g. IASI, see Resources), as there are many aspects of the client/therapist interaction that cannot be explained within a single text.

BodyReading

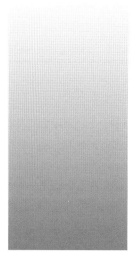

3

Before doing any treatment with a client there must first be some form of assessment. By this stage you will have taken a case history and received a lot of information from the client regarding their medical and structural histories and checked that this form of treatment is safe and appropriate for them. (See Appendix 2 for contraindications.) Traditionally fascial release work employs visual assessment of standing posture and a simple gait analysis. Gait assessment is better conveyed in a class or via our video course (see Resources). In this chapter we will introduce the standing assessment, viewing the client from all four sides (and occasionally down from the top), to gain a picture of their skeletal relationships.

Argument can be made that standing in stillness only gives a limited picture, and that is true. In practice the client could, and should, be observed in movement, particularly any form of movement that appears to be giving cause for concern or is of importance within their lifestyle. Standard movements to view could include walking, bending in each plane of movement, reaching and, of course, breathing. With the limitations of space and two-dimensional images afforded by this book, the myriad variations in range and quality of movement are impossible to portray – so it is from necessity rather than desire that we restrict ourselves to standing pictures and postural analysis.

Our aim with the structural approach to fascial release is to help the client's skeletal alignment via adjustment of soft tissue length and freedom, following the tensegrity view of the body outlined in Chapter 1. We therefore hope to induce the client to 'relax into length' and find easy expansion throughout their whole structural system. This will allow the bones to 'float' more easily within the tissues, aiding joint alignment and function. It also carries other benefits, such as allowing more efficient cellular function (Ingber 1998), and even helping to provide the structural substrate for emotional and psychological balance (Maupin 2005).

BodyReading is both an art and a science that requires time and practice to mature, and the samples we give here are by necessity relatively straightforward and clear. We recommend practicing both the observational skills and the vocabulary outlined below as frequently as necessary to allow them to become natural. As you progress, otherwise boring moments in public places such as queues or airports become laboratories for further development of your seeing skills.

The Five Stages of BodyReading

Our standing assessment protocol has five stages:

1. **Describe** the *skeletal relationships*.
2. **Assess** the *soft tissue* pattern that creates or holds the pattern in place.
3. **Strategise** – develop a *story* about how and why these elements are interrelated, and create a strategy for the order in which those elements will be worked.
4. **Intervene** – do your *work* (in practice this may be a few strokes, a session, or even a series of sessions), and,
5. **Evaluate** – when any given intervention is complete, *reassess and re-evaluate*. This can be done palpatorily, or by having the client stand or perform a particular movement. Did the work have the desired effect? If so, what next? If not, why not? Do you need to change your approach to that area, or is there another area that needs freeing first?

A Positional Vocabulary

To describe these patterns, we need a vocabulary. Though many such vocabularies are in use in different therapeutic professions, four words suffice: *Tilt, Bend, Rotate*, and *Shift*. Though at first it may seem limiting or confusing, once practiced a bit this vocabulary can be used to create a quick sketch of the client's structure, but will also bear the weight of the most detailed inter-segmental analysis – coupled with the standard descriptors of right/left, anterior/posterior, medial/lateral, inferior/superior, and so on.

By using Tilt, Bend, Rotate and Shift, we avoid using polysyllabic Latin terms that can be daunting for the client to hear when they do not necessarily understand the medical jargon. It could be disconcerting for the client to be told their back pain is due to a 'rotoscoliosis', rather than a 'series of rotations and bends in the spine'. So by using common terminology that is intuitively understood, we avoid creating a power differential between ourselves and the clients – yet we can still easily communicate the client's pattern among practitioners from a wide range of backgrounds.

Commonly used professional terms such as *pronation* to describe the feet or *protraction* of the shoulders can be so general in their nature as to give little information about the precise bony relationships, which are a complex array across a number of joints. By using Tilt, Bend, Rotate and Shift, we can accurately describe the position of each bone relative to its neighbor. This gives us much more information about what is happening to the soft tissues which may be holding that pattern. 'Protraction' may lead to a generalised protocol that hopefully works; 'an anterior tilt in the scapula coupled with a lateral rotation of the humerus' leads to precise soft tissue releases.

1. Describe

Tilt

A tilt is defined as a deviation from the vertical alignment. It is named from the top of the structure and the direction in which it moves – left, right, anterior, or posterior. Examples can include a right tilt of the head, a left tilt of the thorax, an anterior tilt of the pelvis, etc. As you can see in figure 3.1, a 'right tilt of the shoulder girdle' implies that the client's left shoulder is higher and the right lower, such that the top of the shoulder girdle leans to his right.

If, as is commonly seen, the pelvis is laterally tilted to, say, the left (left hip lower, figure 3.2), the lumbar spine will usually bend back to the right to render the rest of the body upright, like a tree growing out of a hill. This would then be described as a 'right bend of the lumbar spine', as the top vertebra (L1) is still tilted to the right relative to the bottom (L5).

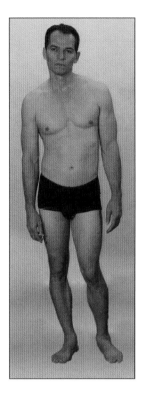

Figure 3.1: In this deliberately exaggerated pose, you can clearly see the rib cage tilt to the right and the head tilting to the left.

Bend

Bends only occur in the spine, and *bend* is used as a shorthand to describe a series of tilts of the vertebrae. We name the direction of the bend according to the direction in which the top of the bend is pointing. If we look at figure 3.2, we can see that a right bend of the lumbar spine is actually a progressive series of tilts of one vertebra on another.

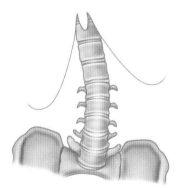

Figure 3.2: A right bend of the lumbar spine showing the relationship of one vertebra to the next.

Rotate

All rotations occur in the vertical axis (when the body is considered in anatomical position), and we name the rotation for the direction in which the front of the named structure moves relative to

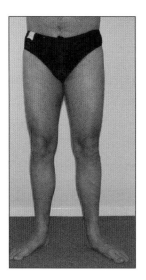

some other part. In simpler words, if you look left, your head is left rotated relative to your feet. Keep your nose and your feet pointed in the same direction, but turn your pelvis around the right. Now your pelvis is right rotated relative to your feet, but your rib cage is left rotated relative to your pelvis. Spend a little time with this if it is confusing; the reward is precise treatment strategies that will get lasting results.

In paired structures such as the humeri or femurs, we can describe them as medially or laterally rotated. Most ballet dancers, for instance, work for lateral rotation of the hip. Many bodybuilders show medial rotation of the scapula.

Figure 3.3: A client demonstrating lateral rotation of the lower limbs.

Plumb lines and grids are commonly used to measure deviations from the gravity line. While obviously useful to determine the weighted leg, such an analysis is severely limited in describing precise intersegmental relationships, and cannot be extrapolated into useful soft tissue strategies.

Shift

The word *shift* is used to describe a translation of the center of gravity of one body part relative to another. For example, in figure 3.4, we can clearly see that the center of gravity of the rib cage has

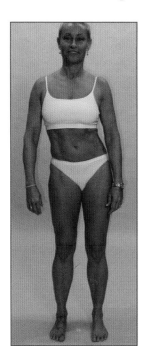

shifted to the right of the pelvis. (It is equally accurate, if not quite as useful, to say her pelvis is shifted left of the rib cage.) For a shift to occur, tilts or bends must be happening in other structures (this woman shows a left bend and then a right bend of the lumbar vertebrae to achieve this dramatic shift). When the pelvis is anteriorly shifted relative to the feet, a common postural fault, there will necessarily be an anterior tilt in the tibia or femur or both.

Figure 3.4: A client demonstrating a right shift of the thorax.

2. Assess the Soft Tissue Relationships

Now that we have the vocabulary to describe the skeletal positioning we need to work out which soft tissue is implicated in the pattern. Our interest is in the soft tissue relationships between adjacent sections, which we will release in the service of balancing the whole pattern.

In figure 3.5a, for example, we can see a mild left shift of the pelvis relative to the feet. Then the rib cage shifts to the right (relative to both her pelvis and the midline) and the head shifts back to the left relative to her rib cage, making it almost neutral to the pelvis. Hopefully you can see that although the head and pelvis are almost in alignment with each other in the photograph, if we brought her rib cage back over her pelvis, her head would then be shifted quite far to her left. Our work will need to focus on easing her rib cage back left to center over the pelvis, while shifting her head to her right relative to the rib cage, all with a view toward easy alignment in gravity over her feet.

Figure 3.5b illustrates a series of anterior shifts: the pelvis relative to the feet, the rib cage relative to the pelvis, and finally the head relative to the thorax. The soft tissue distortion between each of these sections will need to be addressed in turn.

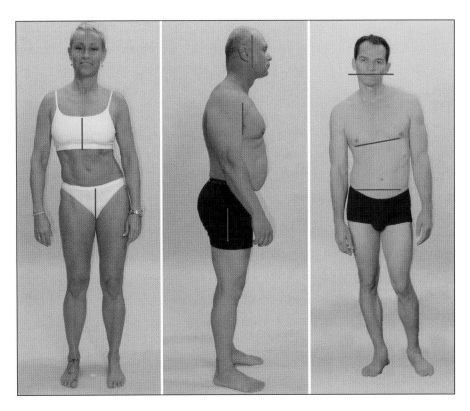

Figure 3.5a, b & c: Here we see three exaggerated postural patterns to allow an easier vision of the skeletal relationships.

Figure 3.5c illustrates a series of tilts, the pelvis to the left and the rib cage to the right. We need to keep in mind that it is the angle of change between these two sections that is important. The lines show how the relationship is measured from the relative angle of difference, not from the horizontal. We take a note of this angle before correcting the issues in his left leg, which could result in balancing his pelvis but creating more tilt (relative to the floor) in his rib cage, such that these tissues below the right rib cage would be crying out for correction. While his neck appears neutral, coming from the right tilted rib cage, it must be tilted to the left to allow the head and eyes to be horizontal. If the tilt of the rib cage is ameliorated, the soft tissue on the left side of the neck would require concomitant lengthening, or the eyes will be tilted, and the client will likely 'reject' the treatment.

By now, it is obvious that, despite the apparent complexity, it is necessary that we read the body relative to itself, not solely to some geometrical template or gravity-based ideal. These general concepts will be fleshed out as we go into detail with each section of the body, as in the key understanding of pelvic tilt, discussed in Chapter 6.

To identify the tissues that have been affected, ask yourself, 'Which two bones have moved closer to each other and what is the tissue between them?' You can then add more detail such as the different levels or depths and the fascial relationships, including which Anatomy Train line or lines might also travel through that area. These kinetic chains can be important if we do not get the desired release or length in an area by working locally. Our attention can then go wider, using the *map* of the myofascial meridians as our guide.

We should also resist the temptation of trying to impose our view of 'correct' posture or what is 'right'. Rather, we should try to view the client as an individual: see where they have wandered away from what God, nature or genes (take your pick or choose your combination) intended for them into what injury, attitude, or upbringing imposed on them. This leads us to our next stage.

3. Strategise

What is it that has taken the client away from that ideal form of themselves? What events in their history have shaped them? What habits have they learnt or what compensations have they developed that have combined to create the shape they now have? And then, how are all of the issues related? Is their anteriorly shifted left shoulder girdle related to the medially tilted right calcaneus? Can you follow the pattern through their body? Does it follow through any of the Anatomy Train lines?

Seeing how compensations travel through the body is a skill that requires time and practice to develop. Starting to build stories around the series of altered relationships in the body as early as possible will help you in choosing efficient treatment strategies. The further into the chain of events you can see, the more you can distinguish primary from secondary effects, the more efficient your treatment pathway can be.

Of course, life is long and complicated, and not every structural compensation you see in a client is likely to fit into one story. But this highly useful if somewhat subjective step allows you to create a coherent and sequenced strategy addressing the specific pattern the client presents.

4. Intervene

Follow your strategy into the practical work of lengthening and freeing tissue according to the techniques that form the bulk of this book. Remember, though, that this is not a collection of techniques, but rather a collection of *intentions*. Each movement is described as if it were specific, precise and absolute. In fact, there are as many variations as there are practitioners and they will all require adaptation to match the variations in anatomy, in tissue type, in pain level, in emotional state and in physical awareness of your client, etc.

The novice will find security in navigating with the guidance of the descriptions; the more experienced bodyworker can strike out for new territory using the descriptions merely as templates for a variety of approaches.

We continually refer to muscle names in the text to locate technique application. Please take it for granted that in each and every case, we intend that muscle name to stand for the muscle and all the surrounding, investing and accompanying fascia. Muscle names, then, are used here as 'postal codes' for the myofascia of that area.

5. Evaluate

After any sequence of interventions – a technique, a series of moves, as session, or a series – you will need to re-evaluate. Have the client stand up, move, and explore moving the area while you take an honest look at what, if any changes have occurred. This step is vital to build and refine our skills, as well as to identify the areas in need of work for our next sequence of interventions.

It also serves to give the client a break, to experience the area anew after the work, to compare it to the other side of the body, or simply to give whatever feedback they feel appropriate. Generally, both the neophyte practitioner and the new client benefit from more frequent reassessment. As you get more experienced, or with a more 'educated' client, your re-evaluations can occur less often.

The BodyReading Process

It is all very well looking at pictures in a book and practicing your new vocabulary on random passersby, but there will come a time when you may need to take the jump (if it is not yet a standard part of your practice) and have your client stand in front of you in their underwear. This can be daunting for both client and practitioner, and we have a few suggestions to make it as natural and as engaging as possible.

1. Use a full length mirror and stand beside and just behind your client, so you are both looking at their image. This puts you 'on the same side' as the client, and is less confrontive than facing the client while making notes (or worse, little clucks of disapproval). Standing with the client emphasizes that this will be a cooperative process; you can both see, assess and experiment with the image in the mirror. This creates the possibility of a discussion of goals for the therapy, what the client likes and dislikes about their body, and their hopes for the work.

When access to a mirror is not possible, you can take digital pictures of the client and have a discussion about them. Both therapist and client can then analyze what can be seen.

2. Notice your first impression, as it can often hold a lot of subtle information. Much of this you may not be aware of or able to verbalize, but often that initial impression can be very rich (as we have a long evolutionary history of acting on first impressions). This information we keep to ourselves, but we note it for future reference, as it may be enlightening later on. It can be something physical, emotional or subtle; it is your impression, whatever aspect of the client that has drawn your attention. It can give us a sense of the essence of a person that we can appeal to as we go through our treatments. A serious nature, a playfulness, an intensity can all be useful allies when it comes to getting some of the work done. (Conversely, some aspects of the client's character may need to be managed in order to focus on the work.)

3. Notice (and communicate) at least three positive aspects with your client first before going into any detail of the BodyReading. We live in a society where so much time, energy and advertising is spent focusing on our faults and failures to live up to the magazine covers that we are only too aware that we are somehow 'wrong' or 'off'. As we like to point out in our trainings there are, however, so many more elements that are going 'right' with their body than are going wrong. By mentioning some of these to your client you not only further engage them in the process but also give them a break from the bombardment of stories of how they need to change.

Noticing positive aspects also brings your attention to the areas that do not need to change, as they are already working efficiently or supporting the client's structure easily. This process puts you in touch with where the client is well-founded and allows you to note where less attention will be needed, making you more efficient. Seeing the areas that are still coherent within the client's structure can give you a sense of how to match the rest of the body to those areas through your work.

In our workshops this is often the first thing that students forget when they come to BodyRead their partners – because we are so focused, not only within society but also as practitioners, on finding fault. Society trains us to see faults, and as practitioners we are eager to 'get it right' in identifying the relevant problems and issues. Pointing out positive features may seem a 'New Age' gimmick and is often forgotten in the BodyReading process, but we urge it upon you as a discipline: in practice it can build rapport quickly, and support the rest of the treatment process.

4. Use the language described above to explain what you see. It is deliberately developed to be as non-judgmental and easily understood as possible, allowing clients to be involved in the process from the beginning and encouraging honest feedback. Having used the mirror in their initial intake, the client will hopefully retain a mental image of 'where they were', and so can compare it to 'where they are now' as the changes take place.

Each of these technique chapters begins with a brief anatomy review, designed to introduce a few relevant concepts for manual therapy, movement, and fascial arrangement. These reviews are not designed to be comprehensive, so please use your preferred anatomy text or those listed in the bibliography as supplementary reading.

The Foot and Lower Leg

4

The unique requirements of human walking and running require a unique foot with major support from the heel. Kangaroos characteristically rest on their heels, but when they hop, they revert to their *paws*. This is the equivalent of us walking on the balls of our hands and feet, an uncomfortable and unsustainable task for us. For most four-legged mammals, rising up on their hind legs – cute in a dog, frightening in a horse – is a very temporary state (figure 4.1).

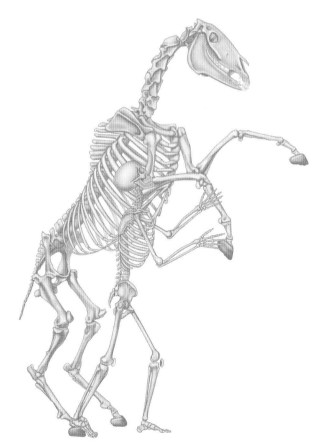

To achieve this, we have two feet that are essentially tetrahedra – three-sided pyramids. This gives us a unique feeling of *grounding*, via our three-legged stool, but it also leaves us in a precarious state of standing, with a high center of gravity and a small base of support. Balance of the feet and the muscles of the lower leg is therefore essential to easy upright standing.

So it becomes our task here to *understand* the arches of the feet. Balance in the arches ensures the correct dynamic between the ability of clients to *ground* themselves – staying connected to the earth in a slightly prehensile way, while still keeping a springy lightness to their step – and with the ability to change direction instantly.

Figure 4.1: Although the bones of the horse and human are very similar, the architecture of locomotion is entirely different.

Understanding the arches rests on three elements: the shapes of the bones, the tension in the plantar tissues, and the balance among the 'puppet strings' of the muscles coming down from the calves. We will look at the three elements in that order, but first we need to put a couple of larger concepts in place.

The Bones of the Leg: As Easy As 1, 2, 3…4, 5

The bones of the leg (and the arm is constructed similarly) can be understood as a progression from the hip to the toes (figure 4.2). In the thigh there is one bone, the femur, and in the lower leg there are two bones, the tibia and fibula.

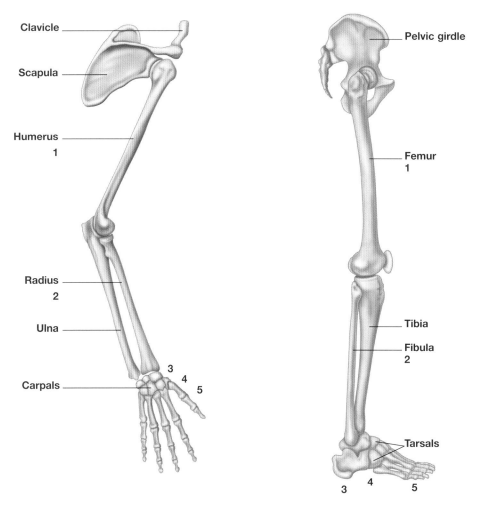

Figure 4.2: The bones of the leg (and the arm as well) go up in number as you get more distal. The single thigh bone is followed by two lower leg bones, followed by three bones in the hindfoot, four bones in the mid-foot, and five in the forefoot.

Of these two, the tibia is the main weight bearer, spreading itself at the top to receive the two condyles of the femur, and resting on the talus below, creating the medial malleolus. The smaller fibula, has its head tucked under the tibia, as if resting under a tree; its lower end forms the outer malleolus, completing the ankle joint.

The next stratum of the foot consists of three bones: the talus, the calcaneus and the navicular. These three bones form the *hindfoot*, and have a complex joint we will discuss below.

The next tier has four bones – three cuneiforms and the cuboid – which together form the proximal transverse arch.

Finally, the five long metatarsals complete this progression from hip to foot. The toes continue this 'five-ness' with fourteen more bones. (The big toe only has two bones, the others usually have three.)

Seeing this progressive complexity from the top down helps us to understand the increasing adjustability of the bones as we move down the leg, and the increasing reliance on the fascial guy-wires we will be working with in Chapter 6.

The Joints: Hinges and Spirals

The joints of the leg have an interesting alternation between a single degree of freedom (producing a hinging motion) and a multiple degree of freedom (allowing rotational motion).

The first joints of the foot, between the various bones of the toes, are all hinges, allowing us to grip the ground. The ball of the foot, the five metatarsophalangeal joints, allows some rotation between the toes and the round metatarsal heads.

The square metatarsal bases allow only a hinging motion (and a very slight but essential one at that). Watch someone walk with a strong, high arch supinated foot pattern, where there is little movement in this mid-foot joint, to see how much the lack of this small give in the foot affects gait in the hip and back.

The next real movement in the foot is at the subtalar or talocalcaneonavicular joint. This joint and the next one up, the tibiotalar joint, are generally thrown into one term, the ankle joint. They are both covered by one ligamentous capsule, such that when we sprain an ankle and cause swelling, both joints are immobilized. But for our therapeutic purposes, we need to clearly distinguish between the joint on the upper side of the talus and the joint below it.

The subtalar joint allows the talus to roll on the rest of the foot or vice-versa; it is a rotational joint. The axis of rotation is not straight through the foot, however, but runs from just inside the big toe to just outside the heel – so this forms the axis of inversion and eversion (figure 4.10).

The tibiotalar joint, or upper part of the ankle joint, is a more straightforward hinge. The top of the talus is mortised into the grip of the bottom of the tibia and fibula, which are 'sutured' together with a strong fibrous syndesmosis. This joint allows dorsiflexion and plantarflexion only.

Since the tibia and fibula are so strongly wired together, only a limited movement is allowed between the two, mostly at the superior end. This rotational movement – equivalent to pronation and supination in the arm – has been shifted into the knee. To feel it, sit with your knee flexed and the ball of your foot on the floor. Swing your heel in and out, and you will feel the medial and lateral rotation of the knee. This can only occur when the knee is flexed, as the knee ligaments prevent such a motion when the knee is extended. (You can still swing your heel in and out with your knee straightened, but then the action happens at the hip joint.)

The regular knee motion is another hinge doing flexion and extension, and the hip is of course a multiple-degree-of-freedom joint, allowing all kinds of movement.

This alternation of rotation and hinging is similarly arrayed in the arm, and in the spine as well. In the latter we find the limited hinging motion of the sacroiliac joint, rotation at the sacrolumbar, hinging in the lumbar, rotation in the lower thoracic area, a hinge in the mid-thoracic vertebrae, rotation in the cervicals, and finally a hinge between the atlas and the occiput.

The restriction of the hinges allows a few muscles to direct the energy of movement very specifically. In other words, if all the joints in the lower arm or leg were rotational, we would all look like Popeye because it would require so many muscles to stabilize them. The alternation of hinge (linear) movements and rotational movements produces spirals of the type we see in a ballet leap or a karate punch (figure 4.3).

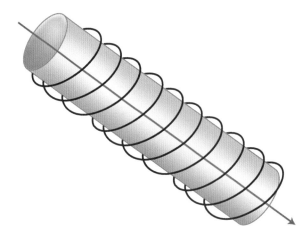

Figure 4.3: Hinges, like the knee or the elbow, create linear, one-dimensional movement. Other joints of various forms, like the hip or the shoulder, allow rotation and multiple degrees of freedom. Combine the two – a linear movement and a rotation – and you get a spiral, seen frequently in dance and martial art forms.

The Arches as a 'Secondary Curve'

Before we deal with the details of the arches themselves, one last concept: the arches are essentially a secondary curve. Primary and secondary curves usually refer to the spine, with the primary curves being those curves that remain from the initial flexion curve present in the foetus and newborn, i.e. the thoracic and sacrococcygeal curves of the spine. Secondary curves develop after birth in response to muscle strengthening: the cervical curve develops as the child learns to lift her head, and the lumbar secondary curve is formed a bit later as the child begins to sit up, developing a balance between the lower erector spinae and the psoas complex.

If we extend this concept 'up', we could include the neurocranium, which comes from the same part of the embryo that forms the spine, and say that the cranial curve is primary, the cervical secondary, the thoracic primary, the lumbar secondary, the sacrococcygeal primary. And to continue 'down': the knee curve is secondary, the heel curve is primary, and the arches are secondary (and if you wish, the ball of the foot is again primary).

In considering this set of primary and secondary waves that alternate up the body from the toes to the forehead, we can note that the entire set is spanned by a myofascial continuity known as the *Superficial Back Line* (from the Anatomy Trains, figure 4.4).

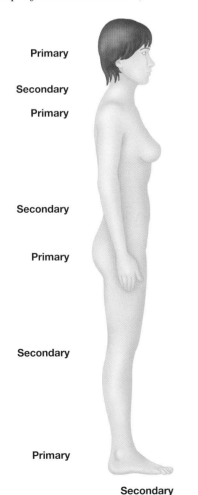

Primary

Secondary

Primary

Secondary

Primary

Secondary

Primary

Secondary

The arches share several characteristics with the other secondary curves in the body: they are concave posteriorly, they act as springs, and they are pulled into being and maintained by the tension in the soft tissues. The primary curves on the other hand, are present from the beginning, and represent the more solid platforms for movement, since they are held in place by the bones.

Figure 4.4: The arches of the foot can be seen as another in a series of secondary curves that alternate with the primary curves on the posterior surface of the body. These secondary curves – including the arches – are less dependent on the bones for their shape, and more dependent on the balance of soft tissue.

The Bones of the Arches

Returning to our area of interest for this chapter, let us explore the three elements that contribute to stable but springy arches. First we will explore the shapes of the bones in each arch (necessary for our understanding, but not really open to much change via manual therapy), then the plantar tissues (which will occupy us for some techniques), and finally, the balance of the musculotendinous guy wires coming down from the calf (which will lead to many powerful arch-maintaining and enhancing manual therapy moves).

The twelve bones of the foot arrange themselves into four discernable arches: the medial longitudinal, the lateral longitudinal, the proximal transverse and the distal transverse (figure 4.5).

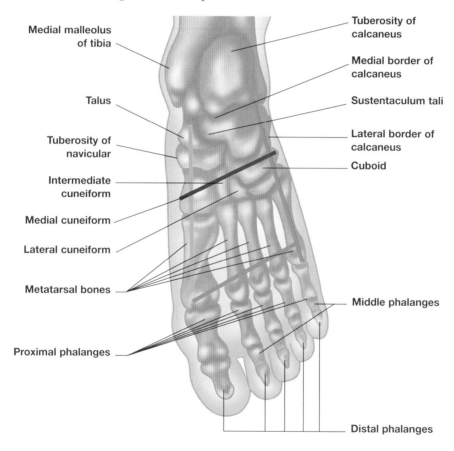

Figure 4.5: The twelve bones of the foot proper hang together to create four distinct arches – the ◼ *lateral longitudinal, the* ◼ *medial longitudinal, the* ◼ *proximal transverse, and the* ◼ *distal transverse.*

The *lateral longitudinal arch* is made up of four bones: the calcaneus, cuboid, and fourth and fifth metatarsals. Taken together, these bones form a good Roman arch, as the cuboid is actually more like a keystone than a cube – narrower at the bottom than the top – so that it stays in place more easily. Dancers call this arch complex 'the heel foot'. Although it clearly bears significant weight in standing, we offer a second image for this complex in movement, which is that it acts as a balancing 'outrigger' to the 'canoe' of the medial arch.

This role is easily felt if you come up onto the balls of both feet. Notice how the weight is primarily taken by the first three metatarsals, while the outer two take far less pressure, but act to help make the constant little adjustments that allow you to stay aloft. Try to shift that weight to the outside of the feet and make the lateral arch take the bulk of the weight, and see how fast you lose balance when the balancing part of the act is required to stabilize enough to bear weight.

The *medial longitudinal arch* rests atop the lateral, starting with the talus, whose rounded head fits into the navicular. This is followed in turn by the three cuneiforms and their concomitant metatarsals. Though this arch bears most of the body's weight, it is not constructed as well as the lateral one in terms of its bony engineering. The first cuneiform in particular, is slightly wider at the bottom than at the top (necessary for walking, but a compromise in support). With the rounded end of the talus, and the slightly dodgy cuneiform, the medial longitudinal arch is subject to collapse, or 'falling', more than its lateral partner.

The *proximal transverse arch* is, like the lateral longitudinal arch, well constructed in terms of the shapes of the bones, comprising the three cuneiforms and the cuboid. The cuneiforms, as the name implies, are wedge-shaped, with the wider part at the top. With tight ligaments underneath binding the bottoms of the bones together, this arch is very difficult to collapse, short of a serious auto accident, or jumping from an airplane without a parachute.

Finally, we come to the *distal transverse arch*, running between the first and fifth metatarsal heads. Here the bones offer us no help whatsoever, since the rounded heads of the metatarsals are only loosely connected with ligaments, and are certainly not arranged to construct an arch. If this arch is functioning, the calluses under the first and fifth balls will be the most prominent. If the arch is fallen, the calluses under the second and third metatarsal heads will be the biggest. Since keeping this arch aloft depends entirely on the strength of the soft tissues, particularly the tone of the adductor hallucis muscle, this leads to our next element, the soft tissues below these arches.

The Plantar Tissues

We have been talking about the foot arches in terms of Roman-style arches, but of course such arches require something solid at either end to tie into, and our feet are self-contained and moveable. The arches therefore, while defined initially by the shapes of the bones, are not sustained from outside the foot, but from the soft tissues above and below.

Taking 'below' first, the plantar tissues sustain the arches by acting like bowstrings under the bow of the arches (figure 4.6). In the case of the proximal transverse arch, the soft tissue component is the set of ligaments traversing the foot between the first cuneiform and the cuboid. Not only are these ligaments difficult to reach, it is inadvisable to lengthen them in any case, since rarely do we find a proximal transverse arch that can be counted as too high. In the case of supinated feet and other patterns known as *high arch patterns*, work on the other three arches and lower leg will suffice.

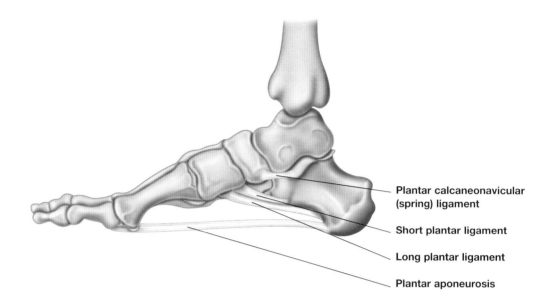

Plantar calcaneonavicular
(spring) ligament

Short plantar ligament

Long plantar ligament

Plantar aponeurosis

Figure 4.6: The plantar fascia acts like a trampoline or bowstring to help hold the arches up and keep the bones from spreading under the weight of the body.

The distal transverse arch, in contrast, is almost entirely dependent on the soft tissue running between the first and fifth metatarsal heads. Although some manipulative work to open these tissues may be required, the principal sustainer of this arch is the adductor hallucis muscle. This needs to have increased tone to support the arch, hence the common prescription to scrunch a towel under your toes or pick up small objects with them. Both of these exercises strengthen the muscles that help support this arch.

The lateral longitudinal arch is supported by the lateral band of the plantar fascia, accompanied by the abductor digiti minimi muscle, which run in tandem from the outside bottom of the heel bone to the base of the fifth metatarsal (figure 4.6). This tissue is shortened in 'fallen arches', visibly so in more serious cases.

The medial longitudinal arch is supported by the main body of the *plantar fascia*, or plantar aponeurosis, which is stretched between the front of the heel bone and the heads of the first and fifth metatarsals, rather like a triangular trampoline. You can feel this structure on the bottom of the feet if you pull your toes into hyperextension; notice how it starts wide at the balls of the feet and narrows to no more than two centimeters or so by the time it reaches the front of the heel.

The short toe flexors lie deep to the trampoline of the plantar fascia and above them is the long plantar ligament and the short but very strong spring ligament, all of which help support the arch system, by preventing the bones from spreading longitudinally. These structures are difficult to affect manually, since they lie so deep.

The Calf Muscles

The final element in the arch system, and the one most amenable to our fascial re-education efforts, is the support offered by the pull of the muscles in the lower leg. These muscles are arranged around the combined structure of the tibia and fibula, and the interosseous membrane that joins them.

These muscles are easily divided into four compartments of two or three muscles each (figure 4.7). We will introduce each compartment, and then show how they combine to move the two ankle joints and provide support (or not) for the three arches.

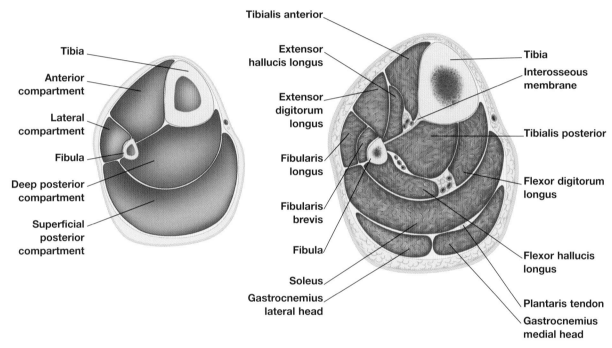

Figure 4.7: The eleven muscles that affect the ankle joints are divided into four compartments by the fascial intermuscular septa.

The *superficial posterior compartment* contains the gastrocnemius, soleus and plantaris muscles. The gastrocnemius and the (very weak) plantaris are the only lower leg muscles to cross and act on the knee, where they act as weak knee flexors, but primarily as leg steadiers. Plantaris is a small muscle, a weak plantarflexor for the ankle, but plays an important neurological role in assessing and adjusting the tension in the Achilles tendon. Below, all three of these muscles insert into the top of the heel, making them strong plantarflexors, or preventers of dorsiflexion. The soleus has a large attachment to both tibia and fibula above, and is a primary postural muscle preventing collapse of the ankle. It also steadies the leg as we move our hands and heads far above the tiny tripods of the feet.

The *anterior compartment* contains the two long toe extensors, which can also play a role in adjusting to the movements of the body above, but have no real role with the arches. The third and largest muscle of this compartment, however, does: the tibialis anterior runs down across the face of the tibia to attach to the joint between the first cuneiform and first metatarsal, which is a weak link in the medial longitudinal arch.

All of these muscles are held down where they cross the ankle by thickenings of the deep investing fascia (crural 'sock') known as the *retinaculae*. These retinacula, often shown as separate and regular structures in anatomy books, are in fact a highly irregular and individualized part of the leg's long outer sock.

The *lateral compartment* lies just lateral to the fibula. It is bounded by two strong fascial septa, and contains two muscles, fibularis longus and fibularis brevis (formerly known as the peroneals – figure 4.8). Both muscles descend behind the fibular malleolus, using it as a pulley. The fibularis brevis makes it only as far as the fifth metatarsal head on the outside of the foot, pulling that bone strongly into the cuboid to keep the lateral arch snug. The fibularis longus reaches under the cuboid (thus supporting the lateral arch) and across the under surface of the tarsal bones to insert into the joint between the first metatarsal and the first cuneiform. This muscle thus tends to pull down on the medial arch, everting the foot. In fact, both these muscles are plantarflexors and everters at the ankle. They are thus preventers of inversion and protectors against ankle sprains.

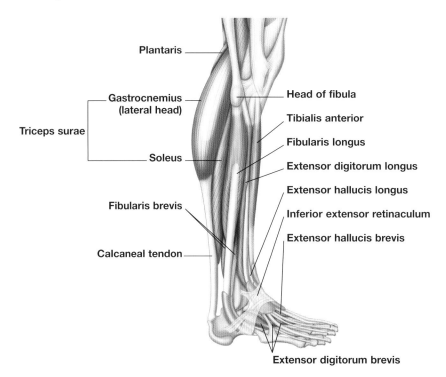

Figure 4.8: From the lateral side, we can see three compartments of the leg: the posterior compartment with the triceps surae, the lateral compartment with the fibularis muscles, and the anterior compartment with the toe extensors and the tibialis anterior.

The last compartment of the lower leg is the *deep posterior compartment*, which lies between the large soleus and the interosseous membrane. The three muscles in this compartment include the two long toe flexors – flexor hallucis longus and flexor digitorum longus – and the very hard to reach but vitally important tibialis posterior.

All three of these muscles pass behind the medial malleolus of the ankle, but only the tibialis posterior uses it as a pulley, passing from there under the medial arch, attaching to most of the tarsals except the talus itself. In this way, the tibialis posterior joins with the tibialis anterior to cooperate in lifting the medial ankle off the floor, maintaining supination and preventing pronation.

The flexor digitorum longus and the flexor hallucis longus cross on their way to the toes, so that when you flex your toes, they tend to come together – probably a left over from when we used our feet to climb trees. Lift your toes and they come apart; flex your toes and they come together, due to the angle of the flexors creating a gripping effect; the same is true for your fingers, by the way.

The flexor hallucis longus additionally works to support the medial arch in a crucial way. If you pull your big toe into hyperextension, you can find the flexor hallucis tendon as a distinct band along the medial edge of the plantar fascia on the bottom of the foot. Put your thumb into the dip created between the Achilles tendon and the back inside of the ankle and then press your thumb forward against the back of the lower tibia. Flex and extend your toe to feel the flexor hallucis tendon moving behind the ankle (careful: the tibial nerve is in there too, so be nice to yourself).

In figure 4.9 you can see how the flexor hallucis longus really goes from behind the tibia to behind the talus and under a piece of the heel bone that reaches under the talus. Thus, this tendon goes right under the major downward weight of the entire upper body. When is the flexor hallucis longus really strongly used, i.e. when would it be tight? At the very moment of push-off, when the weight coming into the medial arch is considerable and the need for support is great.

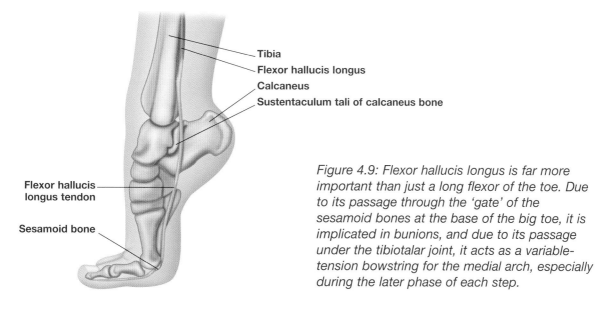

Tibia
Flexor hallucis longus
Calcaneus
Sustentaculum tali of calcaneus bone

Flexor hallucis longus tendon

Sesamoid bone

Figure 4.9: Flexor hallucis longus is far more important than just a long flexor of the toe. Due to its passage through the 'gate' of the sesamoid bones at the base of the big toe, it is implicated in bunions, and due to its passage under the tibiotalar joint, it acts as a variable-tension bowstring for the medial arch, especially during the later phase of each step.

By combining these muscles, we humans get a number of unique ways of supporting our arches, despite the considerable weight coming down on such small bases of support. Each of these combinations can contract or relent from moment to moment to reinforce the arches.

The *sling*: The tibialis anterior and fibularis longus combine to make a sling under the medial and lateral arches. Tautness in the sling supports both of these arches, and the proximal transverse arch as well. This is a well-known and important sling, and both muscles and this sling are contained within the Spiral Line in the Anatomy Trains map. If the fibularis longus is too short and the tibialis anterior overstretched, this contributes to a collapsed medial arch, or everted foot. If the tibialis anterior is too short and the fibularis longus overstretched, the tension will contribute to the tendency toward a supinated, high arch foot.

The *ice-tongs*: The tibialis anterior and fibularis brevis both pull posterior and superior and medial from their lower attachments at the base of the first and fifth metatarsal respectively, and thus draw these two bones into the tarsum of the foot, preventing the collapse of the tarsus.

The *fireman's carry*: The tibialis posterior reaches out nearly to the lateral side of the foot from the medial side. The fibularis longus reaches over to the medial side of the foot from the lateral side. Together, they pull the medial and lateral sides into each other, reinforcing the proximal transverse arch as well as both longitudinal arches.

These slings reinforce the actions of the individual muscles – the fibularis muscles in supporting the lateral arch, the tibialis muscles in supporting the medial arch, and the flexor hallucis longus in supporting the medial arch.

Muscle Actions

Let us look beyond the arches to the general actions of the lower leg muscles on the foot. These actions depend little on where the muscles begin in the calf or where they end on the foot, but rather on the precise point where they pass the ankle joints. We have previously noted that the ankle is two joints: the upper tibiotalar joint that dorsi- and plantar flexes, and the lower subtalar joint that inverts and everts.

The axes of these two movements are shown in figure 4.10, and the placements of most of the tendons are likewise shown in this figure. Any tendon posterior to the axis of the tibiotalar joint acts as a plantarflexor; any tendon anterior to that line acts as a dorsiflexor. Any tendon medial to the axis of inversion-eversion acts as an inverter, and vice-versa.

Tendons that are located farther away from the axis of movement exert themselves more powerfully.

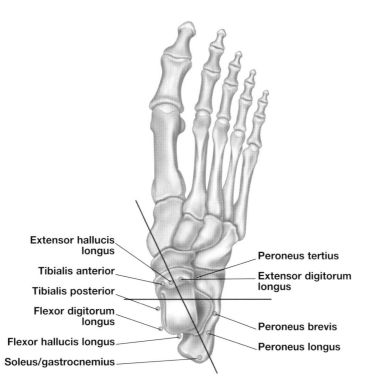

Extensor hallucis longus
Tibialis anterior
Tibialis posterior
Flexor digitorum longus
Flexor hallucis longus
Soleus/gastrocnemius

Peroneus tertius
Extensor digitorum longus
Peroneus brevis
Peroneus longus

Figure 4.10: The placement of tendons around the ankle joint determines their action in plantar- and dorsiflexion and inversion-eversion. The farther away from the axis the tendon is, the more powerfully it acts in that movement. Thus, the tibialis anterior is a powerful inverter and dorsiflexor, while the extensor hallucis longus can dorsiflex, but is a weak inverter.

Note that the axis of eversion and inversion is not exactly along the longitudinal axis of the foot. This leaves the calcaneal attachments of the triceps surae firmly in the inverter column. These powerful muscles retain tone even when relaxed, and this accounts for the phenomenon that most people have their feet inverted when they lie down on your treatment table. Thus, the best way to read foot posture is with the client in standing with the knees relaxed, not supine on the table.

Finally, we should note that all muscles can be considered to work from origin to insertion, or vice-versa, from distal attachment to proximal attachment. That many muscles have names and primary descriptions in the books that emphasize the proximal to distal action should not deter us in our examination of muscle function from both ends.

This is especially true in the lower leg, where often enough the foot can be moved on the lower leg, but more often, these muscles are stabilizing the lower leg on the planted foot. Thus, we could see these eleven or so muscles reaching up from the foot to stabilize various aspects of the lower leg (and thus the whole body above) on the stable foot. The implication of this in figure 4.10 is that the dorsiflexors become the 'preventers of plantarflexion'. The inverters become the 'preventers of eversion'. When seeking stability and grounding in our clients, this reverse action of the muscle is what we need to remember.

BodyReading the Foot and Lower Leg

As discussed, the foot is the underpinning structure that can determine much of the integrity for the rest of the person's body. We can aid that relationship by seeing how the many joints are aligned, and checking the support for and by the arches. We would like to see a foot that is free and adaptable, supporting the transfer of weight through its complex to the ground as we move through the world.

Have a look at your client's feet. Where do they point in relation to the pelvis? Are they rotated medially or laterally? If they are, look at their knees. Do they go in the same direction? Often you will see torsions in the knee, when the femurs appear to be rotated in one direction and the tibia and fibula in another (we will deal with this in Chapter 5 but it can be important to see now). If the femurs, the tibia and the feet rotate in the same direction and to the same degree then the problem is more likely to be at the hip; but we need to find the source of the problem by checking down through each joint in turn.

We need to keep a determined eye for the source of any rotation or variation from 'normal'. Obviously we would be missing a large part of the picture if we were to see the foot rotated and immediately accept that the hip rotators need work. With a lateral rotation of the foot relative to the tibia then we need to think of working with the fibularis muscles (particularly the fibularis brevis) and the lateral band of the plantar fascia, as the base of the fifth metatarsal will be drawn closer to the calcaneus. Even the tissue of the abductor digiti minimi may need to be lengthened to help correct the lateral pull on the forefoot.

A lateral rotation of the foot can often result from a weakness of the medial longitudinal arch, as once the inside of the foot loses some of its integrity, it can overstretch the medial tissue, making the lateral aspect relatively short.

When looking at the arches we need to be clear which bones are tilting; a lower arch can be due to a medial tilt of the calcaneus, or further forward in the foot with the talus and medial cuneiforms, even the metatarsals can be tilted. Different patterns will lead to different strategies, as each pattern will involve a different set of fascial supports, which we will address below.

You can get a sense of the integrity of the arches by looking at your client in standing, but also have them bend their knees slightly to check the tracking of the joints and to watch how the arches adapt to the movement. Having them walk can eventually be very informative, but it takes practice to see exactly what is happening in the mechanics, as it all happens so fast. We recommend starting by just doing it as part of your intake and see whatever you can see, trusting that gradually the small points will become more obvious with time and practice. Watch what happens when the foot is in the air and what happens on heel strike, and notice how the feet roll through and push off, looking for any excessive tilts or rotations. How does the foot relate to the knee? Does the knee swing in or out or straight forward? What you then have to work out is which of the many guy ropes for controlling these movements may be fascially short or muscularly weak, as this will give you your strategy.

If we look at our model in standing (figure 4.11), we can see that she has less support on her right medial longitudinal arch than her left, though it too is allowing the whole foot to tilt medially. The right foot is more laterally rotated than the left. This may be in part causing the apparent right tilt of her pelvis, the right side of which seems lower than the left. There is also some torsion at the knee, where the femurs appear medially rotated relative to the tibias.

When we see her come forward into a deep knee bend (figure 4.12), we can see how this translates, with the right knee in particular tracking medially, and both tibial tuberosities coming over the hallux rather than along the line of the second metatarsal. You may also be able to see how this affects the tracking in the ankle joint.

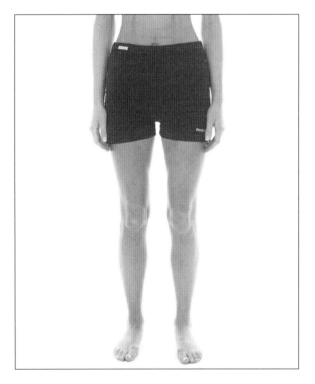

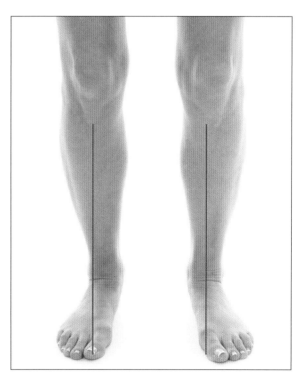

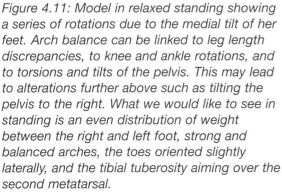

Figure 4.11: Model in relaxed standing showing a series of rotations due to the medial tilt of her feet. Arch balance can be linked to leg length discrepancies, to knee and ankle rotations, and to torsions and tilts of the pelvis. This may lead to alterations further above such as tilting the pelvis to the right. What we would like to see in standing is an even distribution of weight between the right and left foot, strong and balanced arches, the toes oriented slightly laterally, and the tibial tuberosity aiming over the second metatarsal.

Figure 4.12: When performing a knee bend, the tibial tuberosities should pass over the second metatarsal, not the big toe as seen here.

We can then take this into our strategy and think of which tissues may be short or long and which direction we could work them. Tibialis anterior and tibialis posterior will be weak and long, their tissue dropped, being overpowered by the relatively short fibularis muscles that have pulled the medial longitudinal arch down (longus) and the base of the fifth metatarsal laterally (brevis). This pattern will be reversed in high arch or laterally tilted feet.

There are many issues involved with the feet and we will look at some more as we describe the techniques below.

Foot and Lower Leg Techniques

Opening the Foot

When approaching work with the foot and leg, get a feel for it. Take the foot in your hands and move it. Move each of the joints, the talar, the subtalar. Feel the relative resistance of the foot as you move it from inversion to eversion, plantarfexion to dorsiflexion, and as you pass each metatarsal past its neighbor. This is not an intellectual process. Let go of thinking about it and simply feel through the movements. It is the beginning of getting to know the client's tissue, to develop a relationship with it, to understand it.

The first few times you do this you may achieve little more than an introduction to the client. But after a few clients you will start to get more and more information, letting you assess where the restrictions or limitations may be, leading you to better, more precise strategies and more direct, more successful interventions.

You can repeat this process with each limb or body part you come to; it is a simple listening process that reveals information and allows the client to relax (when done just enough and not too much!). This instruction will not be repeated for each section within the book, so keep it in mind if you find it useful – or if you ever find yourself thinking 'What the heck could I do next?' It can give you a chance to gather new information, leading you somewhere new (and can also satisfy that need, sometimes distracting, to feel that we are always doing something for the client).

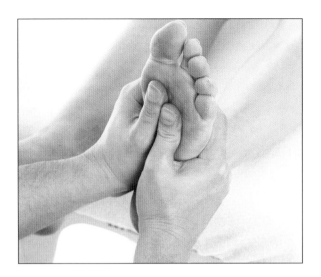 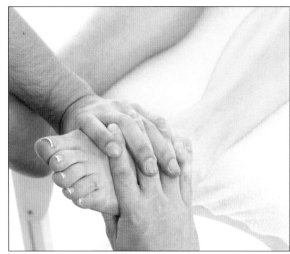

Figure 4.13a & b: Taking a firm hold of the foot with both hands, thumbs controlling the sole, can allow you to assess each joint of the foot and even areas as high as the hip joint. Take the foot slowly into all the various movements open to it, 'listening' for subtle variations in where it can or cannot go.

Clearing the Ankle Retinaculum (SFL)

Earlier we talked of the retinaculum being part of the 'long sock' of the leg. This 'sock' is the deep investing layer, the third skin of the body, a fascial container and supportive structure.

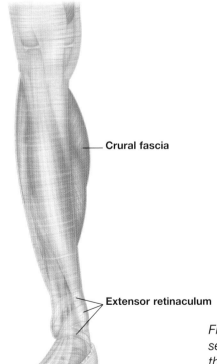

— Crural fascia

Extensor retinaculum

Figure 4.14: The retinaculum is often shown as a series of discrete structures, but in reality it is a thickening within the deep investing layer. This is the continuous covering of the body, and it is given different names in different sections. In the leg it is called the 'crural fascia'.

The tendons crossing over the anterior aspect of the ankle can often become bound into the folds of the back of the retinaculum, restricting their free passage. In order to release them, the therapist can engage into the deep investing layer, of which the retinaculum is merely a thicker element, and lift it superiorly as the client plantarflexes and dorsiflexes her foot to move the underlying tendons. Work from the base of the toes to a few centimeters above the ankle joint.

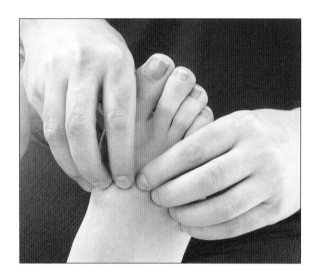

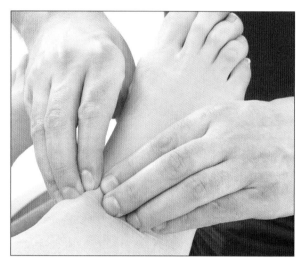

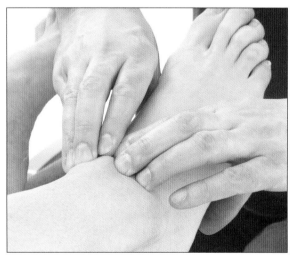

Figure 4.15a, b & c: This is an ideal area to practice the palpation of the deep investing layer, sinking your way down through each of the strata. Feel the different quality as you press through the skin, through the adipose layer, and feel the resistance as you reach the deep investing fascia. Try locking your contact at each of these layers on the dorsum of the foot. Feel the difference in quality not just of the tissue but in the control you have of the foot and toes as you move each layer in turn. If you have a sensitive partner, one used to bodywork or in tune with their body, have them give you feedback as you build your specificity and skills.

The freedom and independence of each layer is important for efficient functioning of all parts of the body, but the foot and ankle seem particularly susceptible to becoming bound because of the many insults to which they can be subjected. Taking time to 'clear' each layer can be very useful after any form of immobilization, such as post-surgery or sprain. Movement can even be reduced down into the layers of the tendosynovial sheaths which surround the tendons in this section. Locking into the sheaths as the client makes the tendons move creates a kind of flossing effect, freeing any restrictions that may have been present.

Freeing the Metatarsal Five

The twenty-one bones of the foot are designed to be adaptive, forming themselves to variations in walking surfaces and footwear. We can lose this ability due to wearing solid, hard-soled or ill-fitting shoes, after injury or insult, or just as a result of walking primarily on sterile, flat, man-made surfaces.

As part of your introduction to the feet, hold each metatarsal just proximal to the heads and pass them by one another in the dorsal-ventral plane, feeling for the changes in relative freedom. The fourth and fifth should be easiest to move, with the restriction gradually building from third and fourth to second and third, with a slight ease between first and second. Any that seem a little more stuck than the others can be worked out by gently mobilizing them in just the same way as for the assessment phase, but they can also be worked more deeply by sinking a fingertip between them to open the affected lumbricals and interossei (the small muscles between the metatarsals).

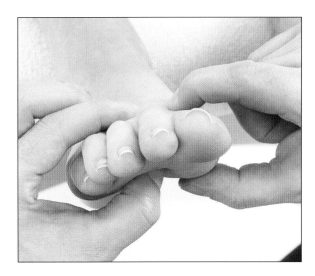 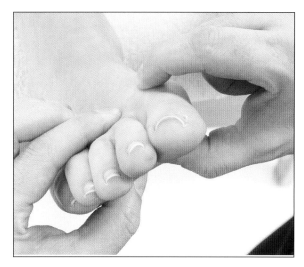

Figure 4.16a & b: Holding each of the metatarsals in turn and passing them alternately back and forth to assess their relationship to each other.

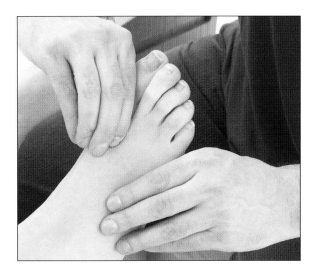

Figure 4.17: Working between the metatarsals to open the lumbricals.

Plantar Fascia (SBL)

This thick and important piece of connective tissue often needs to be worked in order to help release the calcaneus and to correct an apparently high arch pattern (figure 4.20a & b), but distortions of parts of the plantar fascia occur in nearly every aberrant foot pattern. This is, of course, a highly innervated area, so working with care and good body mechanics helps maintain friendly relations with the client in this potentially painful site.

The client can lie either supine or prone with their feet over the edge of the table, allowing the foot to move freely through plantar- and dorsiflexion. Sit or kneel at the foot of the table and work along the lines of the tissue with your knuckles. Your shoulder, elbow and point of contact are all on the same vertical plane, allowing your bodyweight to be transferred directly through your bones, easing the pressure your soft tissue.

The movement is achieved by locking your shoulder, elbow and wrist, sinking your bodyweight forward into the tissue on the sole of the foot, and then lifting your shoulder to create a downward angle on your knuckles. The lift of your shoulder comes not from elevation but from rocking your bodyweight onto the opposite ischial tuberosity. This style of body-use (creating a stabilizing force further up the chain rather than pushing at the site of contact) allows your stroke to be softer and therefore easier to receive in what is often a tender, sensitive area. You should experiment with this technique as much as possible, as it not only helps your client but is maximally ergonomic for your own body as well.

Cover the area with two or three passes along slightly different lines, making sure you also address each of the separate slips that attach to the metatarsal heads. Ask the client to plantarflex and dorsiflex to help release and educate the tissue. It is always easier to use your bodyweight in this way by coming over the top to work downward, rather than pulling the tissue up. So by turning the client into a prone position, you can then alter the direction and still maintain ease in your body mechanics.

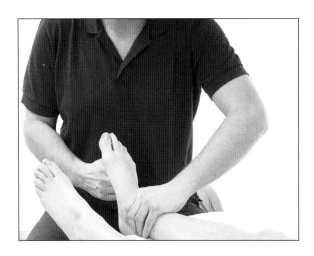

Figure 4.18: Here we see the vertical alignment of the point of contact, wrist, elbow and shoulder, which allows the easy transfer of body weight into the tissue.

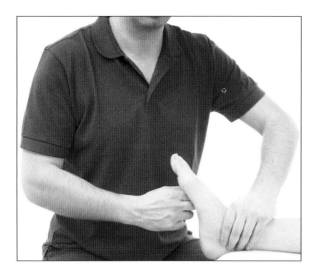
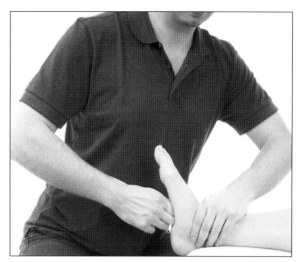

Figure 4.19a & b: Raising the shoulder by lifting the trunk creates the downward angle, giving a strain-free contact.

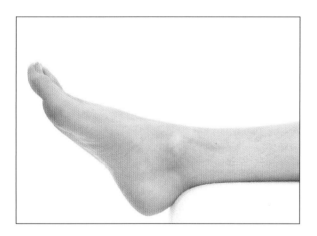
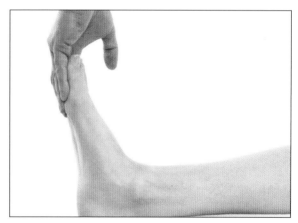

Figure 4.20a & b: Short plantar fascia can give the appearance of a high arch pattern, but when the ball and heel of the foot are put on the same plane we can see that the arch is normal.

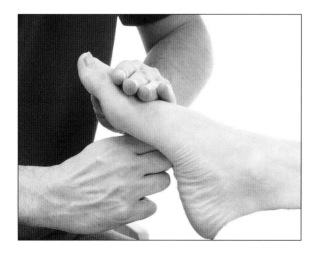
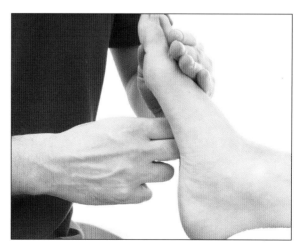

Figure 4.21a & b: To access the deeper layers of the plantar tissue, begin your engagement with the foot slightly plantarflexed to ease the superficial tissues, and then have the client slowly dorsiflex their foot (figure 4.21b).

Lateral Band of the Plantar Fascia (LTL and SBL)

This lateral band can be involved with both lateral rotations of the foot and fallen arch patterns, as it runs from the calcaneus to the base of the fifth metatarsal, holding those two landmarks closer together.

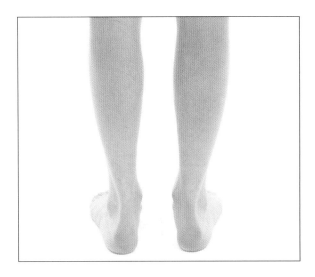

Figure 4.22: Here we see how the foot with a medial tilt of the calcaneus tends to also create a lateral rotation of the foot relative to the tibia.

Lateral rotation of the foot is often seen in combination with a fallen arch (medial tilt of the tarsals). If we are to correct the tarsal position we will have to ensure the fifth metatarsal base is able to move away from the calcaneus to allow the foot to straighten.

Have the client in side-lying, with the foot to be worked on uppermost. One knuckle can be used along this line of tissue, which is running directly between the two palpable bones of the calcaneus and the base of the fifth metatarsal. Note that these bones are up a centimeter or two (half an inch) from the floor – it does little good to work on the very tough padding under the heel.

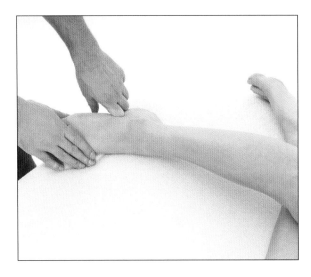

Figure 4.23: One-handed elongation of the lateral band.

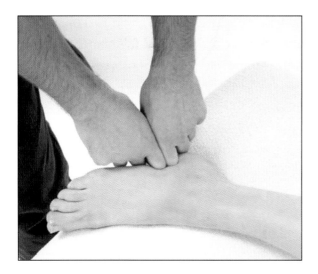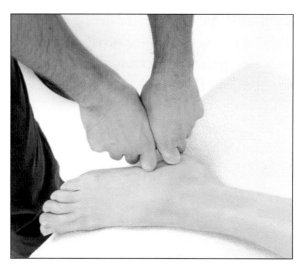

Figure 4.24a & b: Double handed elongation of the lateral plantar fascia. Note how the sides of the fists are together to create a rolling movement of the hands, pushing the knuckles apart.

If space allows, use both hands, pressing the sides of your fists together to push apart the knuckles of your index fingers. The fibularis brevis also attaches to the base of the fifth metatarsal, and so can also be worked as shown above to help create more length between it and the lateral calcaneus.

Freeing the Heel (SBL)

When much of the client's bodyweight is in front of their lateral malleolus it can create extra tension in any of the tissue passing around the back of the calcaneus, which is how the plantar fascia leads the Achilles tendon as part of the Superficial Back Line. This can conspire to push the heel forward into the joint, leading to an apparent loss of length of heel in comparison to the amount of forefoot. This is a phenomenon analogous to the calcaneus being an arrow, with the taut tissue passing behind it taking the role of the bowstring 'firing' it forward into the foot.

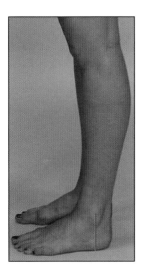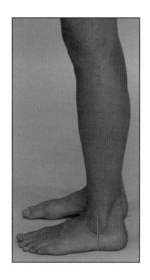

Figure 4.25a & b: Close up comparison of a short (a) and normal (b) heel.

If we are to be successful in moving the bodyweight back over the center of the tripod of support of the foot, we must first provide more support at the back; otherwise the tendency will be to return to the seemingly more stable anterior position.

Lengthening the plantar fascia (figure 4.24) is one method, and time can be taken applying pressure on the anterior aspect of the calcaneus waiting for the tissue to release a little further, but let us also address the tissue surrounding the calcaneus.

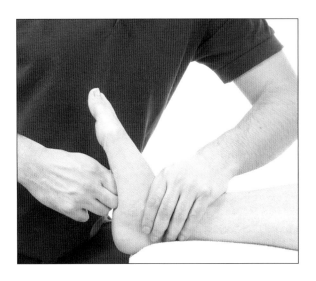

Figure 4.26: Applying pressure with the knuckle on the front of the calcaneus – using a 'soft knuckle' to engage the anterior aspect of the calcaneus and wait for the supportive tissue around it to release it posteriorly.

Working either side of the ankle, the knuckles of the index fingers can be used to free restriction in the tissue approaching the heel, coming down each side from the Achilles tendon, from the malleoli and from the forefoot. With each successive pass the client can reach down with their heel from the hip to create more space.

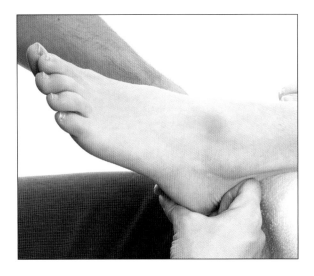 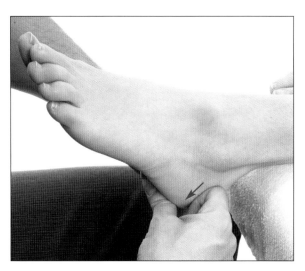

Figure 4.27a & b: Engage the tissue anterior to the Achilles tendon and draw it inferiorly. The stroke finishes at the inferior aspect of the bone not on the fat and below the calcaneus.

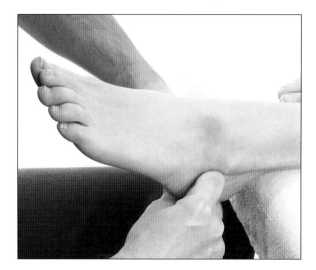 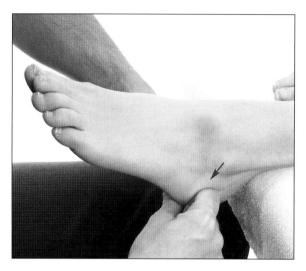

Figure 4.28a & b: Starting slightly below the malleoli to avoid the nerve, draw the tissue back and down toward the calcaneus.

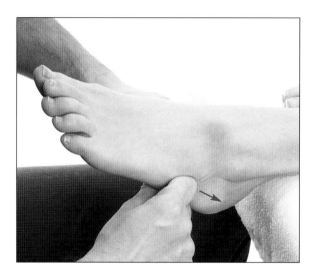 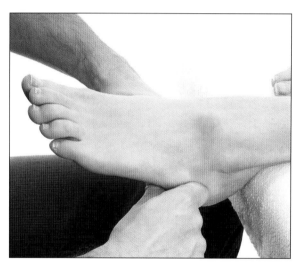

Figure 4.29a & b: Working through each angle surrounding the heel at 0, 45 and 90 degrees respectively.

Other tissues may need to be released before the heel fully moves back: the gastrocnemius and soleus, the hamstrings, possibly even the sacrotuberous ligament or erectors, any of the elements of the Superficial Back Line. The myofascia on the front of the body may also require lifting before the pelvis rests over the feet more evenly. Even a tiny freeing or backward movement of the heel can make a big difference in the support offered by the foot to the rest of the body.

Working with the 'Puppet Strings' of the Feet

Figure 4.10 shows the placement of each of the tendons of the leg muscles as they cross the two planes of the ankle joints. Now consider those two lines of action like the control dowels of a puppet, the tendons being the strings to move the marionette of the feet.

Can you see that by lifting one side you will drop the other? The plantarflexors will antagonize against the dorsiflexors, and the inverters against the everters. By keeping this image in our heads we can visualize the intentions for each of our strokes, particularly in terms of balancing the arches and the actions across the subtalar joint. For example, in the case of a low medial longitudinal arch, we would want to lift and strengthen the muscles on the medial aspect of the subtalar joint line, dropping and loosening the lateral everters. We can help create this by working the tissue in the appropriate direction.

The standard approaches to each of the myofascial units of the leg are given below, but it will be necessary to alter directions or emphasis depending on the pattern that presents with each client.

Releasing the Anterior Compartment (SFL)

Following our general pattern of clearing the superficial tissue prior to delving into the deeper tissues, we want to initially open and assess the myofascia containing the three muscles of the anterior compartment. Using the fist of your outside hand, engage the tissue of the anterior compartment. Often this portion requires lifting, helping to draw up on the inside of the foot, assisting the medial longitudinal arch. The direction of your stroke is therefore most often upward, toward the head.

It could be combined with work on the medial aspect of the tibia by using the other fist simultaneously. If you choose to attempt this, ensure that you engage only into the deep investing fascia, not pressing into the periosteum covering the bone, which will be very uncomfortable for your client.

Both single- and double-handed techniques can start just above the ankle and focus at the level of the crural fascia, engaging the retinaculum and listening for the amount of freedom between them and the underlying tendons. This is aided by having your client's feet over the edge of the table (figure 4.31) and asking them to slowly plantar- and dorsiflex their feet. You can use one hand to guide their movement, particularly if you want to retrain their movement pattern, maintaining their joints as close to neutral as possible rather than allowing them to deviate into supination or pronation.

Carry your stroke all the way along the front of the leg to just below the top of the tibia, around the level of the tibial tuberosity. Adjust your pressure and depth of connection accordingly as you approach this bonier area.

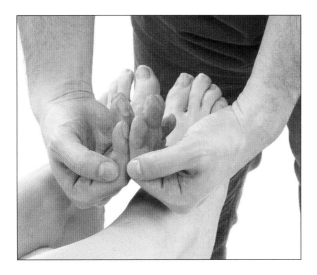

Figure 4.30: Place your hands in a 'rooftop' shape to match the contour of the front of the leg.

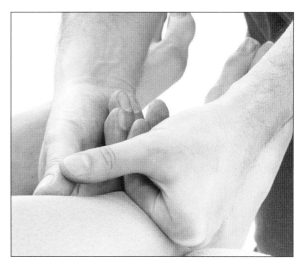

Figure 4.31: Using soft fists, engage the tissue on both the anterior surface of the tibia and the anterior compartment.

Tibialis Anterior, Extensor Hallucis Longus and Extensor Digitorum Longus (SFL)

In order to get deeper and more specific to each of these muscles, you can use either your fingers or knuckles. Because of the density of the tissue in this area, we would recommend using the more stable knuckles, but possibly even an elbow.

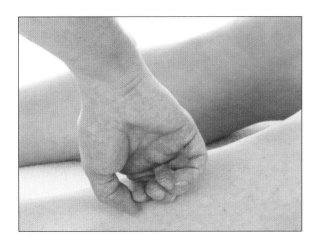

Figure 4.32: A deeper contact can be achieved by using the knuckles, internally rotating the arm and applying a force down through the arm, forearm and wrist.

Using some of the information gleaned from your first pass along the crural fascia, you can now focus on the whole length of the muscles and/or pay extra attention to the areas where you feel restriction or unusual density. The ulnar surface of the internally rotated arm can work along the whole length of the tissue. Return with your knuckles or fingers to deal with the undifferentiated sections of any of the muscles.

The movement for the client is again dorsi- and plantarflexion, though certain aspects of the tibialis anterior may also benefit from asking them to use some inversion and eversion. If you feel for how the tissue opens (or not!) under your contact as they move, then you can gently guide their foot with your free hand in the direction that gives the best challenge to the shortened tissue.

An important area to check along this line can be the gap, or lack of it, between the tibialis anterior and the tibia. Clients presenting with shin pain often have the muscle tacked onto the bone and require it to be cleaned away to give some independence between the two structures. This seems to be of great benefit in the short term, but recurring symptoms can often be an indication of arch and ankle issues, so be sure to assess their gait or refer them to someone who can.

Lateral Compartment and Fibularis Muscles (LTL)

Balancing the medial arches and freeing the fascial septum between the fibularis muscles and the soleus are two of the main structural indications for working the contents of the lateral compartment. You can work up or down along the fibularis longus, forming a continuity of intent with the work performed on the tibialis anterior to either lift or, less frequently, drop the medial longitudinal arch.

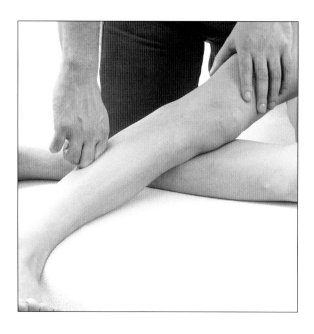

Figure 4.33: Using the knuckles or fingers, you can follow either the line of the fibularis muscles or work in the septum posteriorly between the fibularis muscles and the soleus, or anteriorly between the fibularis muscles and the anterior compartment.

A precise and controlled contact is necessary due to the wiry, strong nature of these muscles. Care must be taken to avoid the peroneal nerve; desist if your pressure produces nerve pain. In order to maintain the focus of your intent on the fibularis muscles, follow a straight line between the lateral malleolus and the head of the fibula.

The client can move the foot through dorsiflexion and planterflexion, inversion and eversion or a circular range of movement.

Posterior Compartment – Gastrocnemius and Soleus (SBL)

The posterior compartment of the leg contains both the soleus and the gastrocnemius, the gastrocnemius being the more superficial and fascially longer of the two, crossing the ankle and knee joints. Both can be affected by a number of postural habits. Whilst they could be worked both superiorly or inferiorly, the more common direction for fascial release work is to take the tissue downward, toward the heel (figure 4.34). To work upward on this tissue, simply reorient yourself to face the client's head, with a similar method and hand position.

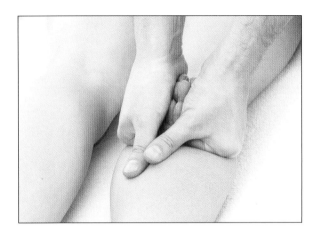

Figure 4.34: Using one or both fists along the posterior compartment (an elbow or forearm can be easily substituted).

The superficial technique utilizes a double soft fist. Keep the focus of the weight on your proximal knuckles (the ones nearer the outside) rather than trying trying to apply force with the middle knuckles nearer the leg's midline, which will require a lot of effort from your finger extensors. Sink into and then beyond the crural fascia. As you work along the back of the leg, ask your client to slowly plantar- and dorsiflex the foot.

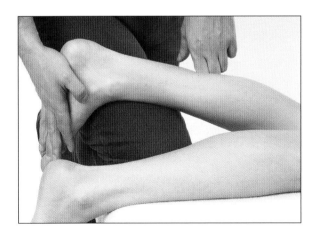

Figure 4.35: To access the deeper layers of the posterior compartment, support the leg in flexion to relax the gastrocnemius and use the knuckles to locate restricted areas. Dorsiflexion is used to release these areas and can be performed actively or passively in this position.

As you are working you may feel deeper and more isolated bands of taut tissue. In order to focus on these, you can support the leg either with your thigh or with a bolster, leaving the client's foot free to move. This serves to relax and shorten the gastrocnemius, allowing more comfortable access to the deeper fibers, which you can then lock into with either your knuckles or fingers. The client's foot can then be dorsiflexed passively or actively, in order to increase the challenge on the engaged tissue.

Deep Posterior Compartment – Tibialis Posterior, Flexors Hallucis and Digitorum Longus (DFL)

This deepest group of muscles of the leg hides behind the tibia, attaching to the back of the bones and their interosseous membrane, making them difficult to get at for the manipulative therapist. Their tendons are easily palpated toward their distal end just before they wrap around the medial malleoli, but where we will get much more release is a little more proximal and where their epimysium is more open and malleable.

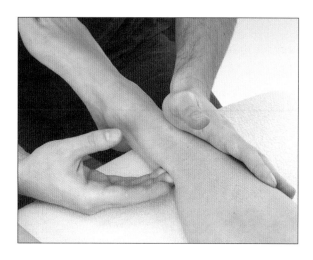

Figure 4.36: Use the lateral hand to push the leg onto the fingers of the medial hand. This allows the contact into the tissue of the deep posterior compartment to be more relaxed and therefore easier to receive. In this position it is easiest to take the tissue superiorly.

In order to get to this portion of the deep posterior compartment, we need to guide our fingers around the medial aspect of the tibia. This is best done by pushing the leg over the working fingers with the supporting hand. This allows the fingers to be more relaxed and thereby easier for the client to receive.

The direction of the stroke is most often upward, helping lift the tissue of this compartment and give some support to fallen arches. Asking your client to plantarflex and dorsiflex their foot whilst maintaining a neutral alignment in their ankle tracking can further assist this by retraining the neural movement pathways.

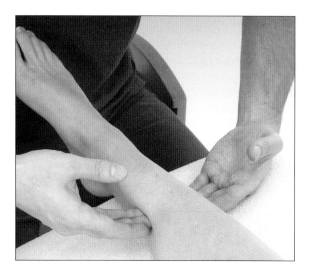

Figure 4.37: With the fingers of the medial hand posterior to the tibia and the lateral fingers in the septum between the fibularis muscles and the soleus, you can engage both sides of the deep posterior compartment.

A deeper stroke involves having both hands work simultaneously on either side of the compartment. The medial fingers once again glide behind the tibia, as above, while the lateral fingers work through the septum between the fibularis muscles and the soleus. Once you sink far enough between these muscles, you should be able to feel the bulk of the deep posterior compartment between the two sets of fingers working medially and laterally. Unless you have a client who is particularly open in this area, your contact will be restricted to the deep investing fascia and epimysium around the group of muscles rather than directly on the muscles themselves, but this level can be worked in the same fashion as above.

It is important to maintain straight wrists through both of these moves. Because of the angle of approach that is necessary it is more difficult to utilize your bodyweight, so a certain amount of upper body strength is required. Keep your elbows wide and slightly behind your point of contact to allow you to lean into the upward stroke as much as possible.

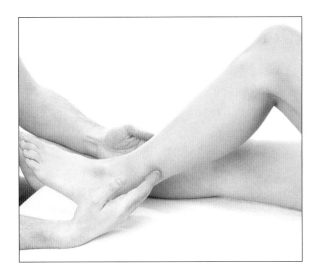

Figure 4.38: An alternative position allowing greater freedom for the client but requiring more stabilization of the thigh.

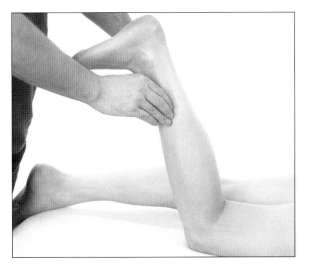

Figure 4.39: Having the client supine can make working in a superior direction easier for you, but because of their orientation it can be less integrating than prone positioning, as it isolates the activity of the foot.

Knee Tracking – Helping Integrate and Re-educate

A useful re-education for the hip, knee and ankle mechanics can be achieved while having your client stand in front of you and first assessing the ability of their knees to track forward over their second toes. Commonly the knees will migrate medially or laterally, depending on the client's individual mechanics. First, ensure that the client's feet are parallel, with the second metatarsals parallel. As they flex their knees forward, the pelvis should stay in neutral, dropping neither into a posterior or anterior tilt.

Once you have taken a reading, hold one thigh just above the patella with your fingers wrapped around the outside of the thigh to hold and control the hamstring tendons. Have the client now repeat the same movement but control their tissue just around and above the knee, so that the patella tracks over the second metatarsal – this is usually quite easy. The harder part comes on the return, where you resist rotation on the way back, holding the leg so it tracks straight back without rotating. You can also engage the tissue around the hamstring tendons with the intention of creating local stretch.

Repeat this process on both legs, and then have the client go through the knee bends unaided but taking care to maintain the correct alignment. The client can be given this exercise to work on at home in cases where the hip and/or knee alignment is challenged.

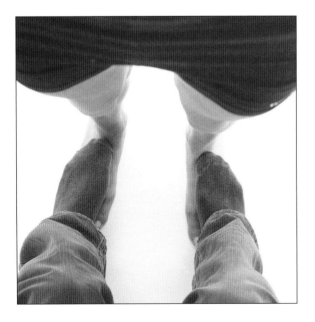

Figure 4.40: Have the client standing in front of you; they can place their feet under yours in order to stabilize them.

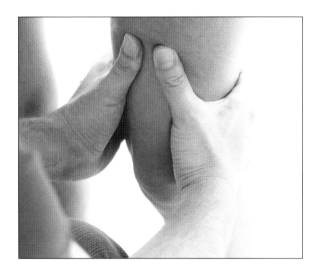

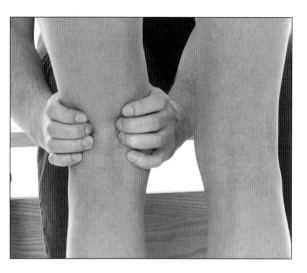

Figure 4.41: The knees may track inside or outside of the second metatarsal, so use your hands to guide them over the second toe.

Figure 4.42: The fingers are wrapped around the back of the knee joint to engage the hamstring tendons, working them particularly on the return.

A useful addition to this technique for those with fallen arches is to contact onto the distal attachment of the tibialis posterior with your fingers as your client stands, giving a slight stimulus and having your client draw their arch up. Your intention is to stimulate the muscle tone, allowing them to recognize and re-own the weakened muscles. All of this will, of course, need to be reinforced with daily activity, awareness and possibly remedial exercises.

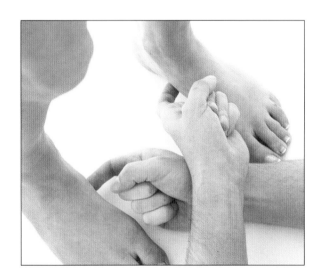

Figure 4.43: To further assist the knee tracking exercise for clients with medially tilted arches, press onto the attachment of tibialis posterior, asking them to draw their arches up from there and to maintain that lift as they perform the knee bends.

The Knee and Thigh

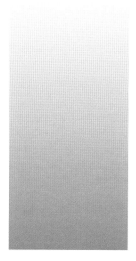

5

The lower leg, while fascially and functionally connected to everything else, is muscularly fairly self-contained. Only three muscles cross the knee joint from below: gastrocnemius and its little friend plantaris both essentially arise from the heel to cross the knee, and the short popliteus participates in locking and unlocking the knee from full extension.

From here on up, we will be making more artificial divisions between the body parts, as more multi-joint muscles blur the boundaries between body segments and consequently the sections of this book as well. Also, we will be 'picking our battles' – choosing a few anatomical points to emphasize among the many marvelous complexities of the body.

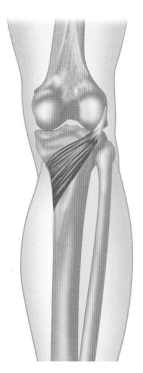

In this chapter, we will talk a bit about the knee joint itself, and then about the long and large muscles that traverse the femur to affect both knee and hip. These muscles give us the strength to run, lift, and coordinate between our foot's foundation and our high-flying spine. In Chapter 6, we will address the hip joint and its largely intrinsic muscles more thoroughly.

Figure 5.1: The little popliteus flexes and rotates the femur laterally on the tibia when the leg is planted.

The Knee Joint

'The knee is an elbow designed by committee', said some wag. The knee sits between the two longest levers of the body – the tibia and the femur – with most of the weight of the body coming down on it (and from various angles in a sporting context).

At first blush the knee seems ill-designed to deal with such titanic and dynamic forces. For starters, the bones do not fit tightly with each other. The femur ends in two rounded condyles, while the top of the tibia is described as a 'plateau'; a fairly flat surface for the femur to land on. This means that there is a certain amount of slide, glide and rotation available at the knee. This makes for a necessary adjustability, but is not so great for stability. All life is compromise, as we stated at the beginning.

Knee ligaments go a long way toward limiting the compromise. The medial and lateral collateral ligaments allow minimal sideways (medial or lateral) sliding of the two bones on each other. The lateral collateral ligament (LCL) is under the iliotibial tract, running from the femur to the head of the fibula, which peeks out from under the tibial plateau. This ligament is not part of the knee capsule, and is very strong and hard to break.

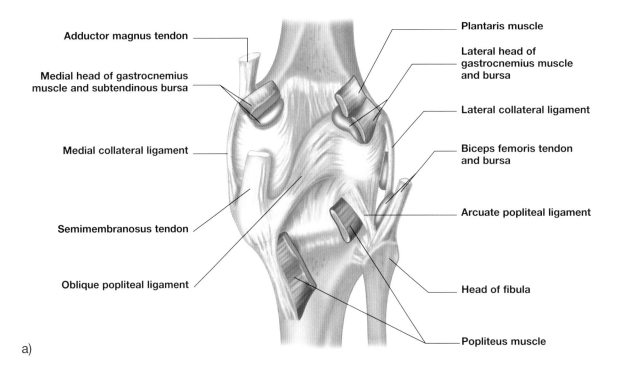

a)

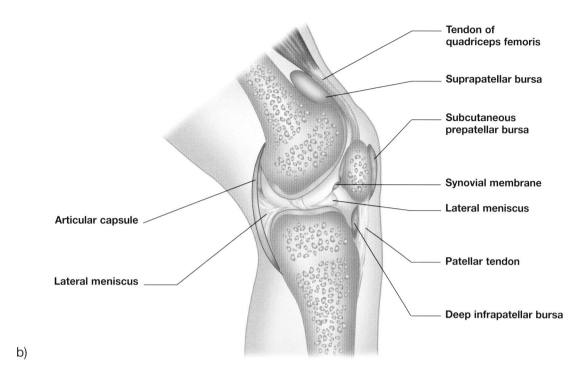

Tendon of quadriceps femoris

Suprapatellar bursa

Subcutaneous prepatellar bursa

Synovial membrane

Lateral meniscus

Articular capsule

Patellar tendon

Lateral meniscus

Deep infrapatellar bursa

b)

Figure 5.2: The knee joint negotiates the forces between the two longest levers of the body – the tibia and the femur; a) right leg, posterior view, b) mid-sagittal view.

The medial collateral ligament (MCL) is part of the knee capsule, making it therefore a bit arbitrary in terms of where we place the scalpel and say, 'This is part of the MCL and this bit right next to it is not'. The MCL, though strong, is not as strong as the LCL, and is therefore more prone to injury. This applies especially with young female athletes, where wider hip joints (on average) and athletic endeavour combine to direct more force into the medial knee. Once weakened, the MCL can be a trouble spot for the rest of one's life, so it is a frequent site for surgery.

The other 'crucial' ligaments of the knee are the cruciate ligaments, so named because they cross in the center of the knee joint. In spite of appearing to be in the middle of the joint, both cruciate ligaments, like the MCL, are simply stronger parts – thick and strong sections – of the complex knee capsule.

The anterior and posterior cruciate ligaments (the ACL and PCL) prevent forward and backward sliding of the femur on the tibia, as well as locking in extension to prevent hyperextension of the knee. There is nothing in the shape of the knee bones or patella that would prevent the knee from flexing to the front – this is the job of the ACL and PCL, which can be made too loose and overstretched by a sustained hyperextended standing posture.

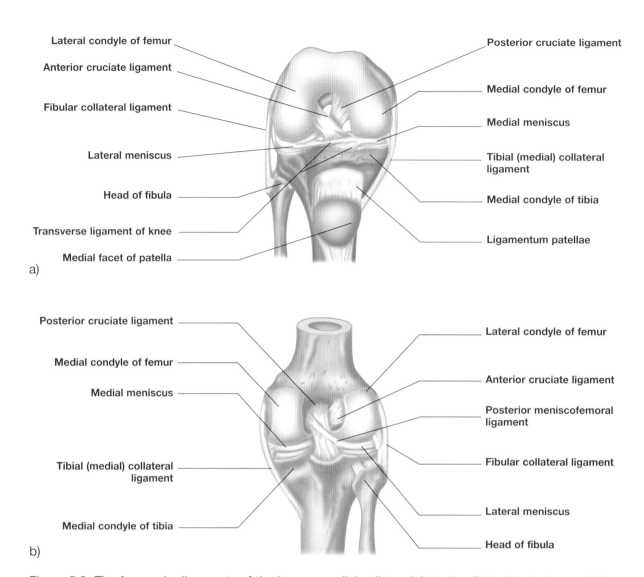

Lateral condyle of femur
Anterior cruciate ligament
Fibular collateral ligament
Lateral meniscus
Head of fibula
Transverse ligament of knee
Medial facet of patella

Posterior cruciate ligament
Medial condyle of femur
Medial meniscus
Tibial (medial) collateral ligament
Medial condyle of tibia
Ligamentum patellae

a)

Posterior cruciate ligament
Medial condyle of femur
Medial meniscus
Tibial (medial) collateral ligament
Medial condyle of tibia

Lateral condyle of femur
Anterior cruciate ligament
Posterior meniscofemoral ligament
Fibular collateral ligament
Lateral meniscus
Head of fibula

b)

Figure 5.3: The four major ligaments of the knee – medial collateral, lateral collateral, anterior cruciate and posterior cruciate – severely limit the side-to-side shearing of the two bones, and limit the front-to-back shearing enough to keep the two bones from sliding off each other in either direction. The cruciates also function to lock the knee from going into hyperextension; a) right leg, anterior view, b) right leg, posterior view.

Tearing or parting of the cruciate ligaments, especially the anterior one, is a not-infrequent football injury – it is, in fact, one injury that sent Moshe Feldenkrais on his quest for healing – and we all feel a little sick when we see a knee bent in the 'wrong' direction. But it is to the ligaments and not the bones that we must look for knee stabilization.

One last point about the ACL and PCL: they are arranged such that they loosen when the tibia is turned laterally on the femur, and tighten when the tibia is rotated medially, or when the femur is turned laterally on the fixed tibia. Many of these knee-compromising injuries take place when the foot and lower leg are fixed on the ground and the upper body is turning into that knee. Examples might include falling downhill over a ski, or that winning twisting backhand shot right after the foot is planted.

Both surfaces on the knee are well covered with thick cartilage, and there are additionally two menisci, semi-lunar cartilages that sit between the tibia and femur, and go a long way toward allowing the two surfaces of these bones to fit snugly with each other. These cartilages lie loosely in the joint (though they manage to have connections with the cruciate ligaments and the medial hamstring tendons). These C-shaped 'rings' of cartilage open when the knee is extended and the flatter end of the femur lies on the tibia, and close when the knee is flexed and the more rounded posterior part of the femoral condyles rest on the tibia.

This arrangement is great when it works, but for all the reasons cited above, these cartilages are subject to being frayed through grinding, or torn or cracked through shock injury. They can even be folded over within the joint as a result of severe twisting.

There is one more unique element of the knee joint that bears mentioning before we go on to the myofascial structures in this region, because it shows what a marvelous piece of design the human body is. The knee joint capsule, in addition to enclosing the area of the joint cartilages and menisci, has two extra 'coves' (figure 5.2). One runs up in the front, under the patella, while the other sticks out the back of the joint and down, under the heads of the gastrocnemius. The capsule cannot go out to either side because of the tight restricting collateral ligaments we described earlier.

When you put your leg forward, you contract the quadriceps. This presses down on the patella, and the synovial fluid beneath it in the 'cove' at first cushions the patella, but is then squeezed through the joint into the back cove. When you push off the foot a second later, you contract the gastrocnemius. This is cushioned against the fluid, but then pushes that fluid back through the joint to the area under the patella. In this way, the joint is lubricated very efficiently at both ends, and the large amount of cartilage in this joint is flushed and refreshed with its 'food', the synovial fluid.

Please note that this mechanism works best in walking, and not so well in running. The best way to naturally care and feed a knee joint is to walk on it – if walking is not contraindicated – as this renews and repairs the cartilage. Walking has about four million years of on-the-job training as a way of healing. This is a solid and concrete example of how it works to renew us.

The One- and Two-Joint Muscles of the Thigh

Depending on how you count, about fifteen muscles could be said to cross the knee. We have already dealt with the ones coming up from the lower leg: gastrocnemius, plantaris, and popliteus. Many of the long muscles that reach down from the thigh to affect the knee are two-joint muscles, i.e. they cross both the hip and the knee. The logic of this arrangement will be our focus as we discuss the muscles of the thigh.

There are five groups of muscles in the thigh: the quadriceps are by far the largest, located in the front, though they spill over onto both the inside and the outside; the hamstrings in the back; the abductors on the outside, tied into the iliotibial tract; the adductors on the inside; and finally a strange little superficial group connected to the pes anserinus on the inside of the knee. We will take each of these groups in turn for a general anatomical description, and then return to the discussion of the balance between one- and multi-joint muscles.

Before we start detailing the individual groups, we should note that if we unrolled the meat off the thigh bone, as one might do with a roast of beef, we would see that these muscle groups have a regular pattern. The muscles on the front and back of the knee come from a narrow attachment at the top and become wider at the bottom. By contrast, the muscle groups on the inside and outside of the thigh start from a wide attachment at the top around the hip, and narrow to a more or less singular attachment below the knee.

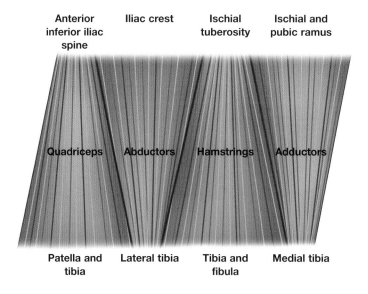

Figure 5.4: The four groups of muscles around the thigh alternate between being wide at the top and narrow at the bottom and vice-versa. The inside and outside muscles are wide at the top; the front and back muscles are wide at the bottom.

By this we can discern that the anterior and posterior muscle groups – the quadriceps and the hamstrings – have more control over the knee working from a stable hip/pelvis. The medial and lateral groups – the abductors and adductors and the odd group attached to the pes anserinus – can be seen to be primarily stabilizing at the knee while being more active in moving the hip. Therefore we will concentrate on the quadriceps and hamstrings and the pes group for this chapter, filling in more about the abductors and adductors in Chapter 6, as part of the fans of the hip.

The quadriceps may have four heads, but it has only one foot: all the tendons converge near the knee into the patella and the bridle of fascia that surrounds and includes it. This bridle attaches all around the front of the tibia, but the heaviest part narrows into a band of fascia that goes from the patella to the tibial tuberosity, a clearly palpable bump at the top of the front of the tibia. The action of the quadriceps then, is through the patella via this band of fascia to extend the knee and kick with the lower leg.

So shall we call this band of fascia the infrapatellar ligament or tendon? On the one hand, it is clearly a tendon, finishing the journey of the quadriceps to their intended target, the tibia, so surely it is a tendon? On the other hand, it is a strong band from the patellar bone to the tibia bone – is that not what we call a ligament?

A further argument for the latter view is that if you put your hand on your leg and rotate the humerus medially to have your elbow over your wrist, your elbow will be in a parallel position to your knee. In this position, it is easy to see that the olecranon of the ulna is in a parallel position to the patella in the leg. By this reasoning, the patella is a 'broken off' piece of the tibia, clearly belonging to the lower leg. That would make the band of fascia joining the two clearly a ligament.

While the discussion might be useful for understanding, there is no definitive answer, other than the fact that whoever created us, He or She has little concern with our nomenclature. This is just a reminder that nomenclature is a human invention, whereas the human body is really not assembled according to such hard-and-fast rules. The rules that shape our body are the much tougher but slower rules of natural selection.

Returning to the quadriceps themselves, these are the most massive muscles of the leg. Three of the heads – the vasti muscles – cross only the knee, and thus restrict themselves to knee extension or resistance to knee flexion. The vastus intermedius runs straight up the front of the femur, attaching all along the way. The vastus medialis and vastus lateralis lie on either side of the vastus intermedius, and wrap around the femur to attach near the linea aspera on the posterior aspect.

The fourth head, the rectus femoris, is a two-joint muscle, also crossing the hip to attach to the pelvis, thus having the action of flexing the hip as well as extending the knee. The attachment point is variable, but the anterior inferior iliac spine (AIIS) is the principal attachment. Some people have a reflected head that curls over the edge of the hip joint; this cannot be palpated. Others have a clear fascial attachment from the quadriceps into the anterior superior iliac spine (ASIS). This anomaly can be very easily palpated when present.

All the muscle fibers within the quadriceps 'aim' toward the patella in penniform fashion. Of course, these are the muscles we primarily exercise when doing squats or other knee extension exercises.

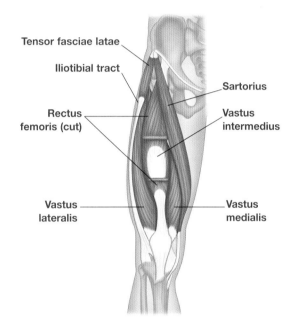

Tensor fasciae latae

Iliotibial tract

Sartorius

Rectus
femoris (cut)

Vastus
intermedius

Vastus
lateralis

Vastus
medialis

We cannot leave these muscles without noting that many gyms are equipped with machines for training the quadriceps that have us sitting while lifting the knee into extension against a bar or weights on the ankle. While this clearly makes the quadriceps stronger and more bulky, we can ask whether such an approach makes the body as a whole stronger or weaker.

Figure 5.5: The quadriceps are the main extensors of the knee (and thus control eccentric flexion of the knee).

Unless you are bouncing your favorite grandchild on your knee, you rarely use the quadriceps in this way. The quadriceps are used in walking, running, kicking, and jumping – all activities we perform standing up, for the most part. Except for two-legged jumping, efficient action of all these activities requires that the opposite hip be stabilized by the piriformis and the other deep lateral rotators.

By doing your quadriceps exercises sitting down, you ensure that the quadriceps are getting stronger, but the neurological connection between the quadriceps strength and the opposite hip stabilization is getting weaker. Those who work to strengthen their quadriceps in this way, are setting themselves up for sacroiliac (SI) joint problems, usually on their non-dominant side if they are not also doing sufficient sport or other exercise to keep the neurological connection strong. 'Fixing' this kind of SI joint pain and dysfunction involves more than a chiropractic or osteopathic adjustment, and more than soft tissue work; it requires some retraining to balance the quadriceps strength with contralateral hip stabilization.

Put your hand on the front of the thigh and you cannot miss the quadriceps. Find the tibial tuberosity first and feel the infrapatellar tendon between it and the kneecap. Palpate either side of the kneecap while your model actively straightens their knee to full extension to feel the connective tissue bridle that surrounds and contains the patella.

Above the patella, the rectus femoris can be felt as a separate muscle running up the surface of the front of the thigh. At the superior end, the rectus femoris can dive under the tensor fasciae latae and the sartorius (which go to the ASIS) to go to the AIIS; though, as mentioned, some recti have attachments to the ASIS, no matter what the anatomy texts say.

The vastus lateralis can be felt along the lateral part of the thigh, lying deep to the iliotibial tract (ITT). Contraction of the vastus lateralis pushes out against the ITT and increases the tension on this band – more on this later.

The vastus medialis can be felt medial to the rectus femoris near the knee; but as you move superiorly, the adductors cover the muscle, which runs deep to them, so that it becomes more difficult to palpate directly. We will take up the palpation of the complex intermuscular septum between these two muscle groups in Chapter 6.

Finally, the vastus intermedius can be palpated between the rectus femoris and the femur. Let your fingertips sink through the rectus femoris gently. You will feel a layer of denser muscle between you and the bone – this is the vastus intermedius.

Turning now to the myofascial complex of the hamstrings on the back of the thigh, we note that there are three hamstrings in classical anatomy, but here we will ask you, for clinical purposes, to consider four.

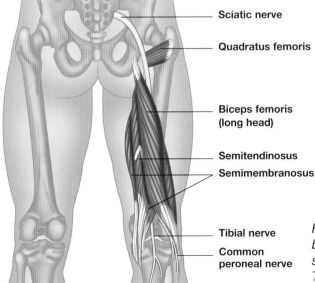

Sciatic nerve

Quadratus femoris

Biceps femoris
(long head)

Semitendinosus
Semimembranosus

Tibial nerve

Common
peroneal nerve

Figure 5.6: The three two-joint hamstrings – biceps femoris, semitendinosus, semimembranosus – fill in the back of the thigh. The hamstrings extend the hip, flex the knee, and control the eccentric flexion of the hip.

Taking the traditional three first – semitendinosus, semimembranosus and the long head of biceps femoris – we can note that they are all two-joint muscles, starting from the ischial tuberosity on the back of the pelvis and attaching below the knee to the lower leg. As such, they all act to extend the hip and flex the knee.

Additionally, the two semis, which go to the medial side of the knee, can participate in medial rotation of the tibia on the femur when the knee is sufficiently bent (flexed). The biceps femoris, attaching to the fibular head on the lateral side of the knee, can rotate the lower leg laterally when the knee is flexed. However, the hamstrings are so often used as stabilizing muscles that we should always consider their eccentric role in preventing or controlling rotation at the knee, extension of the knee, and flexion at the hip.

To find their common proximal attachment, lie your model on her belly and place your palm on the back of the thigh, so that your fingertips lie on the medial part of the gluteal fold. Explore up from here – a little wider on women, narrower on men, generally – to find the ischial tuberosity (IT). Have your model flex her knee and press her heel onto your shoulder or some other resistance to feel the hamstrings pop into tension. In this way, you can feel clearly that the hamstrings attach as a group to the posterior side of the IT. If your model will allow, you can feel the fascial continuity up onto the sacrotuberous ligament that goes superiorly from the IT.

At the distal end, the two semi tendons can be felt on the medial side of the popliteal fossa behind the knee, whereas the single strong tendon of the biceps femoris can be felt on the lateral side. Another interesting palpation is to see how far up the thigh the medial and lateral hamstrings are able to work separately. From the popliteal space between the two sets of tendons, work your fingertips up the thigh. The muscles will come closer together, but you will still be able to insert your fingertips between them.

By comparing various clients, you will find that some people maintain a separation halfway up the thigh or more, whereas in others the medial and lateral hamstrings join fascially a mere couple of inches above the knee. Those who use a lot of side-to-side movement, such as skiers, footballers, and African dancers, will usually have (or benefit from, if they have not) good separation between the medial and lateral hamstrings. Runners, for instance, who always use the full set of hamstrings together, will have less need of such separation.

There are multiple strings and sheets of fascia within these muscles, as their names imply, as well as chronically tight muscles in our fast-paced, gotta-get-ahead world, that can all relent in the face of your skilled work on them.

Turning now to the putative 'fourth hamstring', we have not yet included the short head of the biceps femoris, which runs from the fibular head to the lower part of the linea aspera on the back of the femur. It is, in fact, incompletely separated from the long head; the muscle fibers of both of these blend into one muscular mass (as do the vastus lateralis and vastus intermedius as well), showing again the limitations of our nomenclature in the face of the body's complexity.

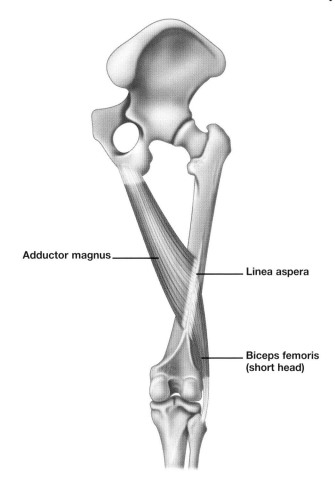

Adductor magnus

Linea aspera

Biceps femoris
(short head)

Figure 5.7: The middle part of the adductor magnus and the short head of the biceps femoris form a fourth hamstring under the other three.

Considered on its own, however, the short head of the biceps femoris is a one-joint muscle that flexes the knee. It is not on its own entirely: the middle part of the adductor magnus comes down to the lower part of the linea aspera, coupling with the short head of the biceps femoris to form a 'fourth hamstring' under the other three. The difference with this construction is that we have two one-joint muscles, whereas all the rest of the hamstrings are single two-joint muscles.

Contract the hamstrings as a group, and you must necessarily exert force to both extend the hip and flex the knee. How does the body control which of these actions is to happen? One way is to control the movement through contraction of the hip flexors or knee extensors, but the other way is via this single-muscle hamstring complex underlying the two-joint hamstrings. The practical application here is that sometimes, when assiduous work on the regular hamstrings has failed to get the release you seek, you will be rewarded by seeking out the underlying middle part of the adductor magnus or specifying the short head of the biceps femoris.

On the outside of the knee, the descending ITT from the tensor fasciae latae and the gluteal muscles (more on this in Chapter 6) act to stabilize the outside of the knee and the lateral collateral ligament. On the inside of the thigh we have a number of adductor muscles, but as none of these cross the knee, we will also take these up in Chapter 6.

The muscles that do cross the knee on the inside are a marvelous little complex of three muscles – the sartorius, gracilis, and semitendinosus. Some anatomist pulled on these three when dissecting, and the three tendons together at their lower end looked like a goose's foot, hence the name *pes anserinus*. All of these tendons help to support the medial collateral ligament, but they are so long that, unless they are fully tensed, their role in supporting is a dubious one.

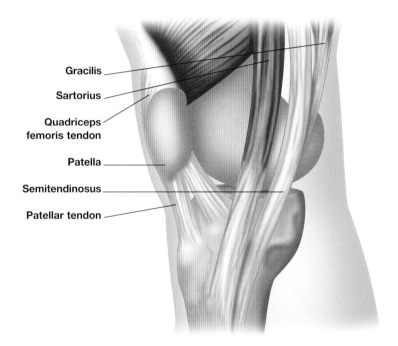

Figure 5.8: The three thin muscles on the inside of the knee – sartorius, gracilis, and semitendinosus – stabilize this 'weak link' to the front, bottom and back of the pelvis.

These three muscles of the pes anserinus go to very different places on the hip: the sartorius goes to the ASIS on the very front of the pelvis; the gracilis goes straight up to the ischiopubic ramus at the very bottom of the pelvis; and the semitendinosus goes to the IT at the back of the pelvis. In this way the inside of the knee can be stabilized to any part of the pelvis. Think of a skater on one leg to see this complex in its stabilizing action.

Thus the muscles of the knee reinforce the stabilizing effect of the ligaments, while at the same time flexing and adjusting the hinge of the knee. Simple but huge, the knee is commanded by some of the largest and strongest muscles in the body.

BodyReading the Knee and Thigh

The lower limb can be comfortably aligned when the feet, knees and hips are in the same vertical plane with a slight flexion present in the knee. We looked at how the foot and ankle joints should be tracking with the tibial tuberosity, and now we can bring the knee into the equation. We would like the tibial tuberosity to be below the center of the knee and the patella nicely placed in the femoral groove. Looking from the side, the most efficient alignment in standing would place the hip joint just over, or just in front of (depending on whom you believe) the lateral malleolus.

When looking at the knee, we can interpret the balance between the medial and lateral hamstrings and the quadriceps. The quadriceps can affect the tracking of the patella within the femoral groove, and the hamstrings' balance can be involved with rotations of the knee because of their attachments onto the tibia and fibula.

Both the hamstrings and the quadriceps also cross the hip joint, and so shortness can also be involved in anterior tilt (rectus femoris) and posterior tilt (all of the hamstrings and adductor magnus). This is dealt with in Chapter 6. We will therefore concentrate on knee patterns for this chapter, though we will include techniques that will also be useful for balancing the pelvis.

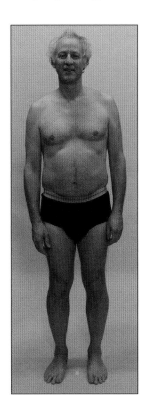

Figure 5.9: This gentleman displays a lateral rotation of both tibias relative to the femurs, particularly on the left, showing a possible shortening of the biceps femoris; but you can also see that the patella is being pulled laterally, indicating an imbalance between the vastus medialis and vastus lateralis.

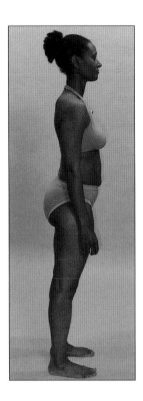

Figure 5.10a: This kind of hyperextension of the knee cannot be held by the quadriceps at the front, as then the profile at the front of the knee joint would be flat. When the tibia and fibula are behind the femur like this then we need to think of the tissue crossing the back of the joint, especially the short head of the biceps femoris.

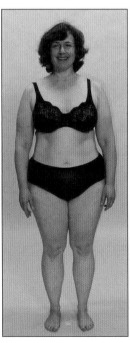
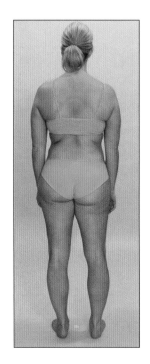

Figure 5.10b & c: When we see these kind of 'X' (medial shift of the knee) and 'O' (lateral shift of the knee) patterns of the legs, we need to address the imbalances between the abductors and adductors (the latter will be covered more in Chapter 6), as they both form another bowstring on the outside and inside of the joint. They can also be tied in with rotations of the femur, causing the profile of the knee to change as the medial condyles become more prominent in lateral rotation to give the impression of 'X' legs and vice-versa for the 'O' pattern. The rotations of the femur will also be balanced through the work of the muscles surrounding the pelvis, and the techniques are therefore covered in Chapter 6.

Knee and Thigh Techniques

Our aim for this section is to balance the forces around the knee joint. As you saw in figure 5.4, there is a wider angulation of possible directions in which the muscles crossing the knee can act in comparison to their proximal attachments, and this can lead to a fairly wide margin of error for the forces acting across this joint.

Releasing Around the Knee (SFL)

As discussed, the fascia from the quadriceps does not all merge into a nice neat line of the tendon we see in many of the anatomy books. Rather, it joins together to form what is called the *quadriceps expansion*, a fascial envelope wrapping over the front of the knee joint and containing the patella within its strong fibrous sheath. It will adapt to the different angles and strengths of pull from the vastus medialis and vastus lateralis, the muscle fibers of which pull on it from oblique angles.

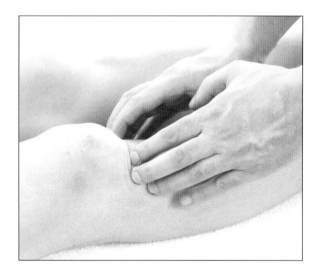
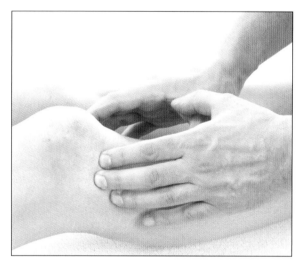
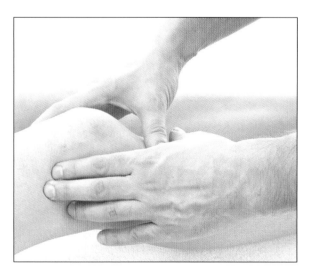

Figure 5.11a, b & c: Use your fingers to encompass the tissue passing around the patella and assess it as the client flexes their knee, feeling for areas of restriction or adhesions, and then focus your contact in that area. Make sure you engage the layer of the quadriceps expansion. If your client experiences a sharp pain, you may be in the deeper periosteum.

By bridging your fingertips over the top of the knee and blending into the level of the quadriceps and then asking the client to slowly flex and extend their knee, you should be able to feel how these different sides relate to one another. Which side is able to open fully? What, if any, is the difference in the quality of the tissue around the knee?

More often than not it will be the lateral aspect needing some extra focus to differentiate the fibers, due to the vastus medialis being less active until the last ten degrees of knee extension (the main exceptions being cyclists and soccer players). In order to release any restricted tissue, simply focus your pressure on that area as the client flexes their knee, lifting it only an inch or so from the table. Any higher and the tissue will tighten too much and push you out.

The imbalance is likely to be more marked above the knee, particularly toward the musculotendinous junction, and can be worked using your knuckles or even an elbow if the tissue requires it.

Pes Anserinus

As a triple attachment site for the sartorius, gracilis, and semitendinosus, the pes anserinus can become quite restricted. It can be found inferior and medial to the tibial tuberosity. With your client supine, engage into the tissue with your fingertips and ask them to slowly flex their knee toward the ceiling, lifting a couple of centimeters from the table. You can simply lift the tissue superiorly or spread it slightly by separating your fingers as the client performs the movement.

Slightly superior to the attachment site, you can work to lift and differentiate the tendons from the underlying tissue. For this movement you can also have your client side-lying, the upper thigh flexed and supported on a bolster as you work with the medial aspect of the lower leg. Ask the client to flex their knee again, but this time use a pincer-type grip with your fingers and thumb to work the tissue free.

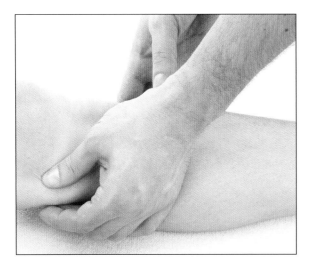
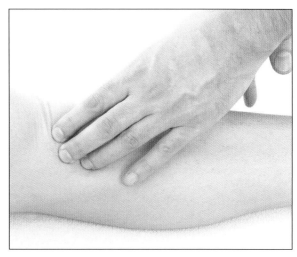

Figure 5.12a & b: Use your fingertips to engage the layer of the pes anserinus and differentiate it from the underlying periosteum and surrounding tissue. Around the medial aspect of the joint, the tissue should be free enough to lift slightly away from the bone.

Quadriceps (SFL)

The rest of the quadriceps will require stronger tools to deal with their bulk. We particularly recommend using a forearm initially, focusing your pressure toward the proximal third of your ulna, but you can change the line of emphasis by rolling your forearm (achieved by lifting or lowering your wrist) to direct your engagement either centrally, medially, or laterally on the thigh.

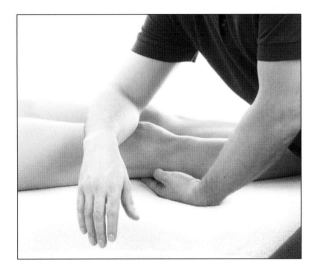 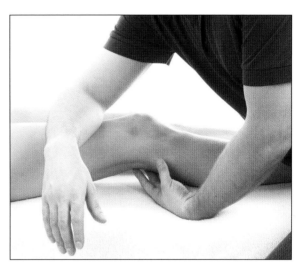

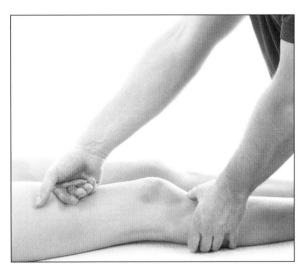 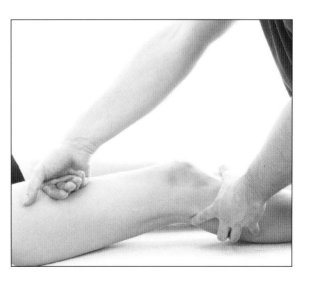

Figure 5.13a, b, c & d: Once the tissue around the quadriceps expansion is eased and balanced, you can then follow further up the thigh with a stronger tool. Releasing the quadriceps with either the forearm or open fist can allow you to cover the larger area, but you can focus on the various aspects by tilting your forearm to engage the rectus femoris, vastus medialis, or vastus lateralis.

If you find a particular line of tension or restriction, then a more sensitive open fist could be used; in the case of isolated areas, even your knuckles would be appropriate.

Remember to ask your client to raise and lower their knee as you pass through the anterior thigh muscles; their movement adds a vital component to the effectiveness of this technique.

Rectus Femoris (SFL)

As mentioned previously, the rectus femoris tendon often bifurcates at its proximal attachment, one section coming to the anterior inferior iliac spine and the other blending into the labrum of the hip joint. Releasing this tendon can be of help in opening the front of this joint and in easing anteriorly tilted patterns. To find the tendon, sink your fingers into the gap between the tensor fasciae latae (TFL) and the sartorius. You can find this hollow by having the client internally rotate their thigh, causing the TFL to contract, and then placing your fingers medial to it. If you strum across, or ask the client to lift their leg, you may feel a thin, ropey tendon.

Engage its tissue with your fingertips and angle your pressure downward and away from their pelvis as you ask them to posteriorly tilt their pelvis (or 'tuck their tail under').

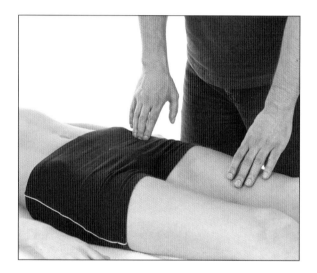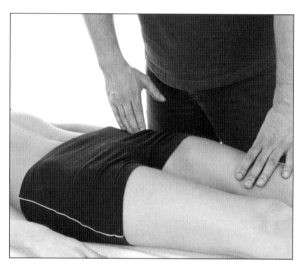

Figure 5.14a & b: Find the hollow between the TFL and the sartorius slightly inferior to the ASIS. To locate the tendon of the rectus femoris, strum across the tissue medial to lateral and you should palpate a thin stringy tendon. To check if you have identified it correctly, ask the client to lift their leg, and the tendon should contract to flex the hip. Engage the tissue inferiorly as the client slowly tilts their pelvis posteriorly.

Hamstrings (SBL)

Before working on the bellies, it can often be useful to release any excess tension in the hamstrings by inhibiting the proximal tendon. Using the elbow of the body hand (i.e. the hand closest to the body), engage onto the tendon, initially just applying compression. Wait for it to release or relax and then, by moving your shoulder superiorly, use your elbow to draw the tissue inferiorly, cleaning the attachment site, giving a very specific opening at the origin of this much-used group.

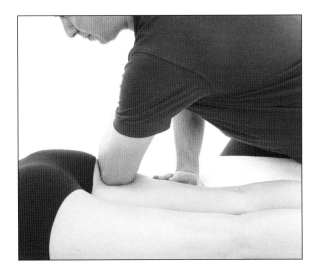
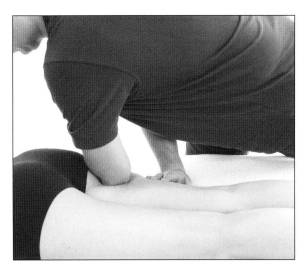

Figure 5.15a & b: Release the hamstring tendon, first applying compression and waiting for relaxation, and then help clean the tissue away from the ischial tuberosity by bringing your shoulder over the top of the contact while you maintain the lock in the tissue of the tendon.

The hamstrings can be lengthened using similar techniques as for the quadriceps. When working either up or down the thigh, it can be easier to use the outside fist for the biceps femoris (lateral aspect of the thigh) and the forearm of the 'body hand' for the medial hamstrings, as this allows for easier body mechanics. The client movement in this case can be to simply press their knee into the table, engaging the quadriceps and hip flexors.

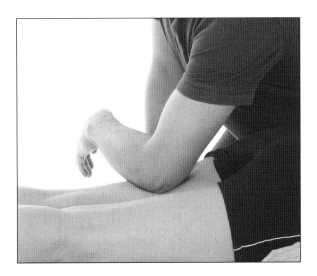
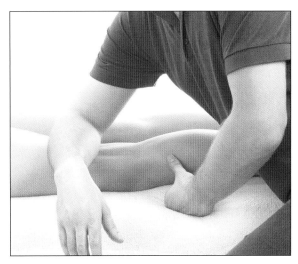

Figure 5.16a & b: The forearm is a useful tool to engage across the span of the back of the legs. Most often the tissue is taken inferiorly along the back of the body to help correct the general pattern.

A more active movement can be to flex the client's leg at the knee and to engage into the tissue, asking them to slowly lengthen it by returning their foot to the couch. This can be done either actively, with the client resisting the pull of gravity, or passively, as you support the leg in a slow return to the table.

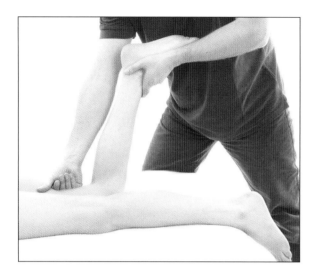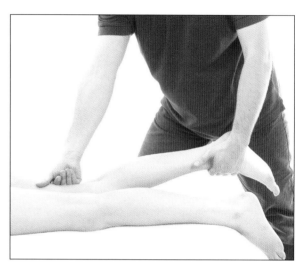

Figure 5.17a & b: A more specific stretch for the hamstrings can be achieved by relaxing the tissue with the knee flexed, locking into any tight or restricted section, and then extending the knee actively or passively.

Separating the Hamstrings (SBL)

Many therapists forget about the knee being able to rotate when flexed. Much of this is controlled by the opposing action of the hamstrings. The biceps femoris will laterally pull the fibula, and therefore the tibia into a lateral rotation. The two semis will draw the lower leg medially. Their ability to do this will depend on the freedom of their respective epimysia, which meet each other in the middle third of the posterior thigh. These 'bags' should be able to glide independently from each other, but often become adhered and may be the source of many hamstring strains.

First, teach your client the necessary movement. With the knee flexed, ask her to turn her leg medially and laterally. Ensure that she rotates the whole lower leg, and does not just wave her feet from side to side, as many will. Once she has learnt the movement, then sink your fingers into the septum between the medial and lateral hamstrings. The contact should be soft; you are swimming your fingers into what should be a relatively open valley. If you are in the right place, you should be able to feel the alternating contractions the client is making by rotating the lower leg in and out on either side of your fingers as they sink. Where the tissue feels restricted, you can tease it open again using both a medial/lateral and superior/inferior prizing action.

The primary area for this work will be in the middle third of the thigh, as the hamstrings will necessarily separate to head to their respective attachments either side of the leg in the distal third, and legitimately merge to form the single tendon attaching to the ischial tuberosity in the proximal third.

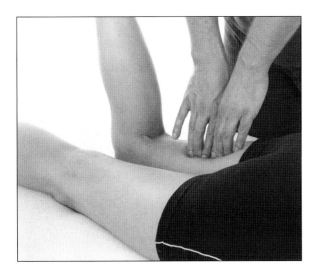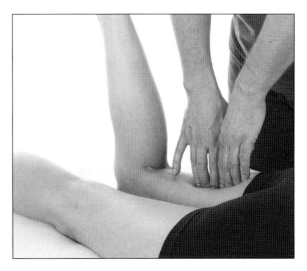

Figure 5.18a & b: The client rotates their leg as you sink into and open the septa between the medial and lateral hamstrings.

Short Head of the Biceps Femoris (SBL)

This section of the lateral hamstring can be important to work and release in many knee issues as it can hold the lower leg in external rotation, perhaps even contributing to hyperextension. It can be accessed using your fingers either side of the more superficial long head fibers, roughly two to three inches superior to the knee joint when the knee is flexed. Sink deep to these superficial fibers of the long head and then push from your chest to bring your fingers together, locking into the deeper section of the biceps femoris closer to the femur. Ask your client to slowly lower their leg toward the table as you engage the tissue superiorly.

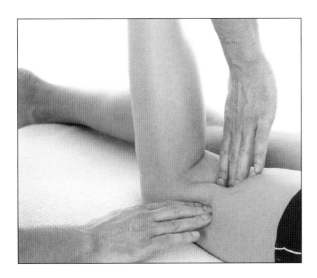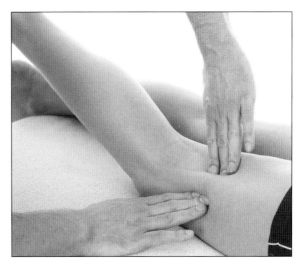

Figure 5.19a & b: Connect into the deep tissue either side of the distal tendon of the biceps femoris, lock in a superior direction, and then maintain your connection as the client slowly extends their knee.

This technique can be performed engaging the tissue both superiorly and inferiorly, as this will isolate the release at either end of the muscle.

Releasing the Gastrocnemius and Popliteus (SBL)

The tissue crossing the back of the knee can be a rich spot for imbalances, and is often considered an endangerment site due to the proximity of the vessels passing through the popliteal space. These can be avoided by wrapping your fingers around the distal tendons, keeping your contact away from the center of the back of the joint. When you sink into the space with the knee flexed, you can access the back of the femoral condyles and lock onto the proximal gastrocnemius attachments and the tissue surrounding the posterior joint capsule. The tissue can be released as the client slowly extends their knee, possibly adding some ankle dorsiflexion to further stretch the calf muscle.

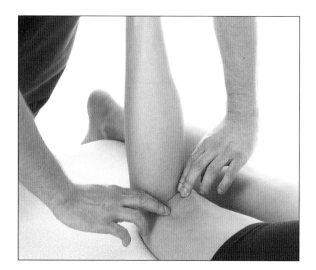
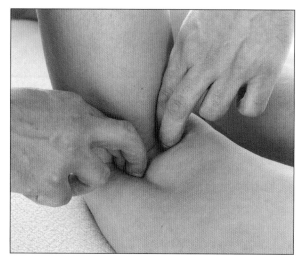
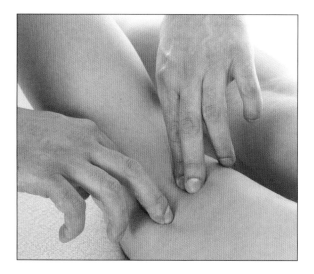
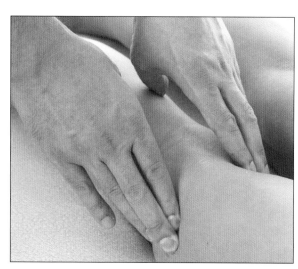

Figure 5.20a, b, c & d: Use the tendons of the hamstrings to guide your fingers to the back of the femoral condyles. Take some of the slack from the skin medially as you enter the space, to minimize the stretch across the popliteal space. Engage the gastrocnemius attachments superiorly and, as the client slowly extends the knee and the tissue tightens, work out over the hamstrings.

This technique should be performed with care and consideration. Ask your client to tell you if they feel any nerve impingement, as you will be working close to the tibial nerve, and the compression and stretch of the surrounding tissue can pull on it. The best way to avoid this feeling of impingement is to 'bring skin with you' as you wrap your fingers around the hamstring tendons, and ensure that during the technique you do not stretch skin between your medial and lateral fingertips. Stinging or nerve pain is reason for you to get out and start again with more slack in the skin.

As the client extends their knee the increasing tension in the tissue will push your fingers out. As this happens, you can then draw the fascia of the hamstrings laterally as your fingers pass either side of the joint.

For a medially rotated tibia, it can also be useful to work the popliteus from the same position. Lock into the distal attachment slightly below the line of the knee joint and emphasize the contact with the fingers on the back of the tibia (it will be the hand working on the medial aspect of the knee; figure 5.20b). In the early phase of knee extension you can also ask your client to rotate the lower leg laterally to gain extra stretch. The limb will naturally return to neutral as it extends.

The Hip

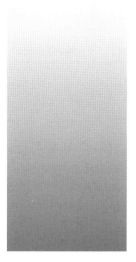

6

Ida Rolf called the hip 'the joint that determines symmetry', because in upright human standing slight differences between the two hips often ramify either down into the legs or up into the trunk. Getting balance around the two ball-and-socket joints is therefore a very important goal for any manual therapist, even when the presenting symptom is higher up or lower down.

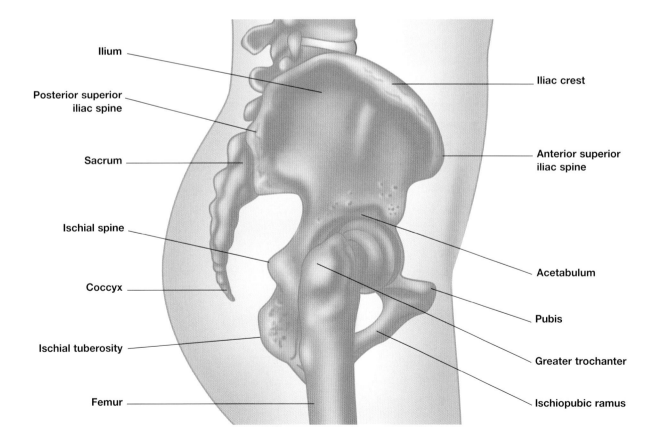

Ilium

Posterior superior
iliac spine

Sacrum

Ischial spine

Coccyx

Ischial tuberosity

Femur

Iliac crest

Anterior superior
iliac spine

Acetabulum

Pubis

Greater trochanter

Ischiopubic ramus

Figure 6.1: Lateral view of the hip.

The hip joint itself is subject to a lot of wear and tear, especially on its cartilage surfaces. The number of hip replacements in both sedentary and active patients testifies to the difficulty the human hip has in staying healthy. Why do our hips not last as long as the rest of us?

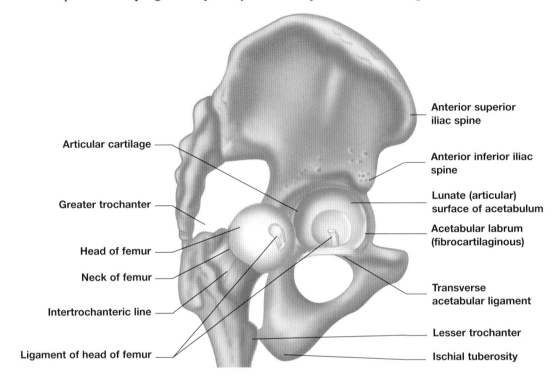

Articular cartilage

Greater trochanter

Head of femur

Neck of femur

Intertrochanteric line

Ligament of head of femur

Anterior superior iliac spine

Anterior inferior iliac spine

Lunate (articular) surface of acetabulum

Acetabular labrum (fibrocartilaginous)

Transverse acetabular ligament

Lesser trochanter

Ischial tuberosity

Figure 6.2: Lateral view of turned out hip.

This joint obviously offers a number of degrees of freedom – flexion, extension, abduction, adduction, circumduction and rotation – which allow humans perched atop these joints to have a variety of movement options. Not quite as obviously, the rounded joint presents a challenge in stability. In order to perform basic movements such as sitting or working with our hands or swinging a bat, we must provide a stability for the heavy trunk that must extend from the slippery ball of the hips to the feet.

To create our various movements, and to prevent collapse or unwelcome movements (i.e., to stabilize), around twenty muscles – large and small, and many of them basically triangular in shape – act to create or prevent movement in a harmonized symphony that changes from second to second throughout our moving day.

We will follow our usual procedure of providing a brief review of the bones, joints and ligaments before making this large number of muscles more understandable as a series of three coordinated fans arrayed around the hip.

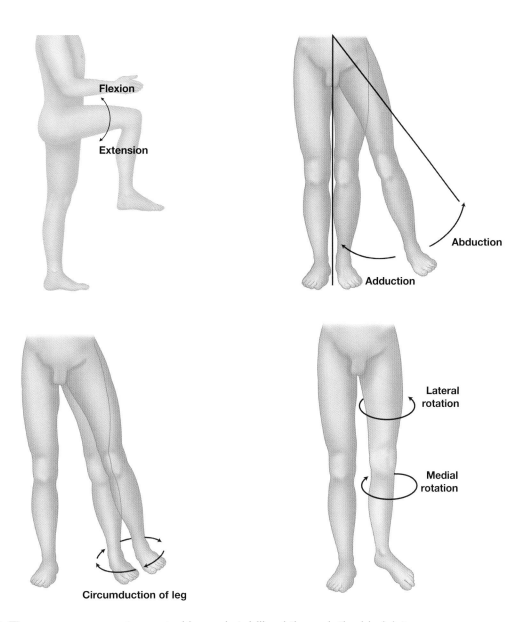

Figure 6.3: The many movements created by and stabilised through the hip joint.

The Bones

The hip joint is the classic ball-and-socket joint. The shaft of the femur sweeps up from the knee to the two protrusions of the trochanters – the greater on the outside for the gluteals, the lesser on the inside for the psoas complex. From the top of the shaft, the neck of the femur angles in gracefully to the rounded head, giving the bone its characteristic '7' shape.

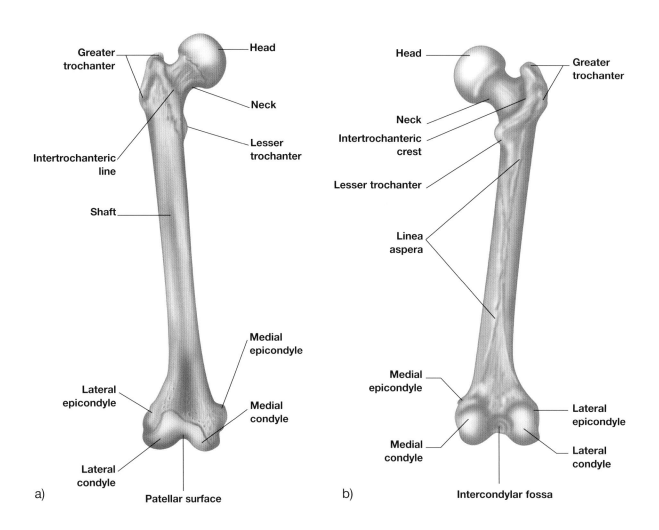

Figure 6.4: Femur of the right leg; a) anterior view, b) posterior view.

The head fits into the acetabulum ('vinegar cruet') of the hip bone, which begins as three bones: the ilium, the ischium and the pubis (figure 6.1). These bones fuse into one (*os coxae* or *os innominatum*, but we will just use 'hip bone' here) by the time a baby is walking at one year old, but the original names survive in the named parts of this bone, e.g. iliac crest, ischial tuberosities and pubic symphysis.

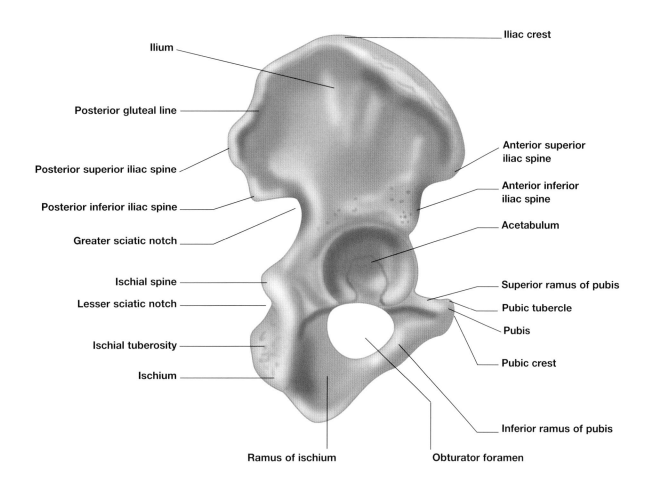

Figure 6.5: Right pelvic bone, lateral view.

Of the prominent and easily palpable bones, the hip bone is the hardest to visualize in three dimensions. The best way to understand the shape of this bone is as a two-bladed propeller. The center of the propeller is right where the head of the femur bears on the top of the acetabulum (which, by the way, is just about where the three original bones of the hip meet).

The upper blade of the propeller is the ilium, with the iliac crest running from the anterior superior iliac spine (ASIS) to the posterior superior iliac spine (PSIS). The bone in the middle of the ilium (between the iliacus and the gluteus minimus) is really quite thin.

The lower blade of the propeller is the ischiopubic ramus, running from the ischial tuberosity (IT) to the pubic symphysis. The 'bone' in the middle of this blade is non-existent, being a hole almost completely covered over with the obturator membrane.

For a propeller to work (although no one is suggesting that the hip bone works like a propeller, just that it looks like one), the blades have to be at different angles, and this is true of the hip propeller as well. Look up or down at a single hip bone, and you will see that a line drawn along the iliac crest from ASIS to PSIS is more or less at 90 degrees to a line drawn along the ramus from IT to pubis.

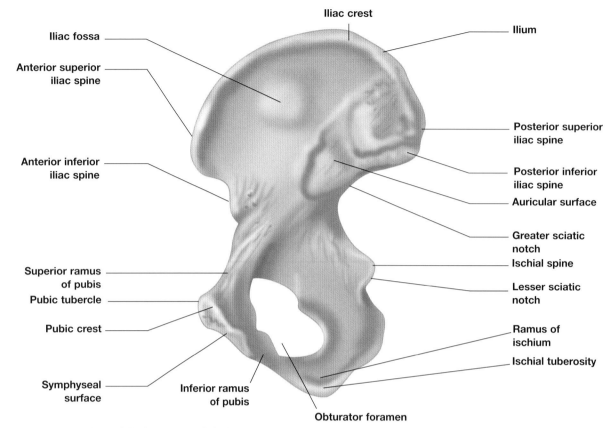

Figure 6.6: Right pelvic bone, medial view.

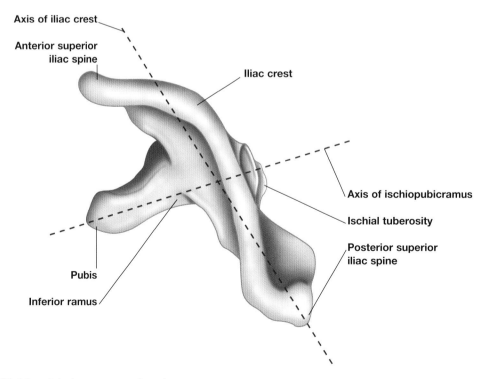

Figure 6.7: Right pelvic bone, superior view.

So, shape a bone into a figure '8' with the acetabulum in the middle, and twist the top and bottom of the '8' to a right angle with each other, and you have the basic shape of the hip bone. The two corners of the pubic bones join at the pubic symphysis, and the two edges below the PSIS join at the sacroiliac joints.

The pubic symphysis is a cartilaginous joint made of fibrocartilage – a strong bridge of collagen fiber embedded in rubbery chondroitin joining the two bones, allowing a little twisting and shearing movement in walking and strong movements of the hips. The combination of the chondroitin and collagen tells us that this joint must resist compression – as in the landing phase of a jump, when the bones are slammed together – and also tension, for example when you swing your leg over a horse. The joint, like all joints around the pelvis, is relaxed somewhat by a relative of oxytocin in childbirth, and thus can be subject to post-partum subluxation.

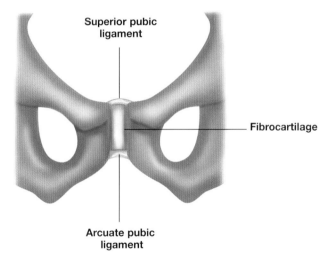

Figure 6.8: Pubic symphysis, anterior view.

The Ligaments

Many ligaments hold the two innominates and the sacrum together in a tightly fitting but slightly moveable manner – a bit like a motor mount linking the legs to the spine, if you will forgive the mechanical imagery. There are three substantial thickenings of the fascial bag around the back of the pelvis that are worth noting. It is also worth noting that whenever we are confronted by a ligament, we need to ask the question, 'What movement does this prevent?' Ligaments cannot initiate movement, only restrain it.

The iliolumbar ligament joins the iliac crest of both innominates to the transverse process of L5 (and sometimes L4). This prevents the hip bones from falling apart when the weight of the upper body comes down through the 'arrowhead' of the sacrum, e.g. when you land on both feet. It also prevents L5 from sliding forward on the sacral table.

The sacrospinous ligament does the same job at the bottom, keeping the bottom of the hip bones from moving away from each other by connecting the lowest part of the sacrum to the ischial spine.

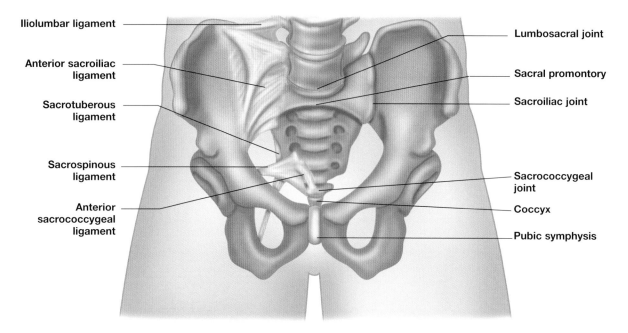

Figure 6.9: Pelvis with ligaments, anterior view.

The sacrotuberous ligament runs more vertically between the hamstrings and the sacrolumbar fascia, joining the IT with the sacrum. This ligament prevents the nutation (anterior tilt) of the sacrum within the hip bones.

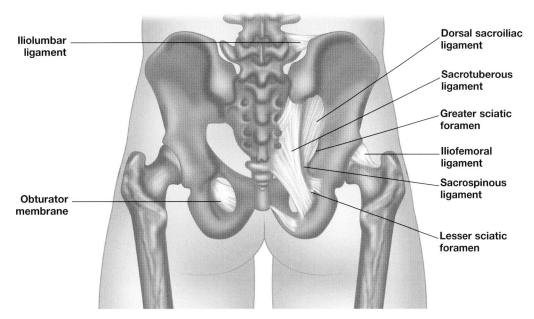

Figure 6.10: Pelvis with ligaments, posterior view.

The sacrospinous and sacrotuberous ligaments divide the space between the sacrum and the ischium into two holes, known as the *greater* and *lesser sciatic foramina*. We will see that each of these holes is filled by one of the muscles of our first fan.

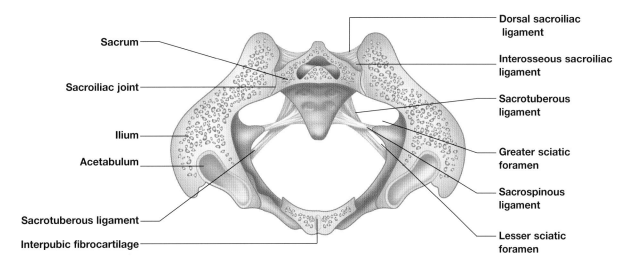

Figure 6.11: Transverse section of pelvis.

The ligaments of the hip joint itself are wrapped around the neck of the femur like a twisted towel. Although there are three ligaments coming from the three bones that originated the hip, they act together as one. The twist is such that when the hip is flexed, the ligaments loosen, and when the hip is extended, the ligaments tighten – especially the iliofemoral ligament in the front just behind the iliopsoas tendon. Thus, if we try to extend the hip joint further beyond our standing position, either by leaning back with the trunk or reaching back with the foot (as in a lunge), we soon run into the limitation created by these ligaments.

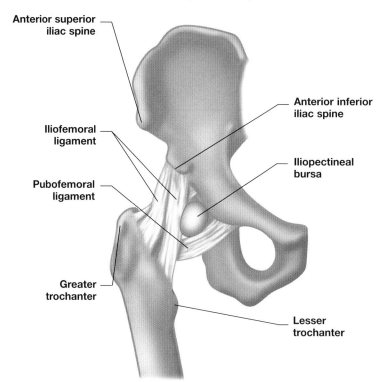

Figure 6.12: Ligaments of the hip joint, anterior view.

In walking, we use this tightness in the extended joint to efficiently transfer the push-off from the foot into forward movement of the trunk. With the knee and hip flexed, we have a lot of play in the hip ligaments and can move freely; with the knee and hip extended, the ligaments in both joints ensure less movement but a more direct transmission of force.

The Muscles

The many muscles of the hip can be understood most easily by seeing them as a set of three interconnecting and coordinating triangular fans around the joint. Each fan has a hub or axis around which it is arranged. Each fan has a rim or outer edge where the wider aspect of the muscle attaches. Interestingly, each fan has what we will term an 'apex' muscle in the middle – a muscle that covers two joints, instead of just affecting the hip. And finally, the transitional muscles between the fans are quadrate, stabilizing muscles.

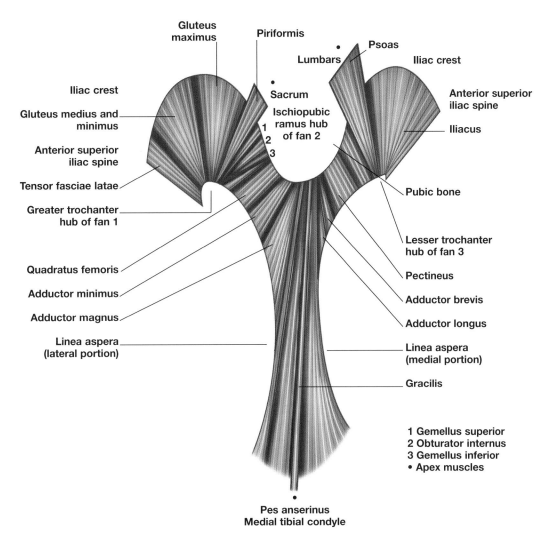

Figure 6.13: Unfolding the series of muscles surrounding the hip joint gives us an insight to the patterns they create and give us the three fans detailed below.

Understanding the muscles of the hip in this fashion allows for a dimensional understanding of hip mobility and stability, and allows us to take on this large meal of muscles in digestible mouthfuls.

We will begin and end at the ASIS, winding our way around one side of the pelvis and taking up each of the muscles in turn, within the context of the three fans as a whole.

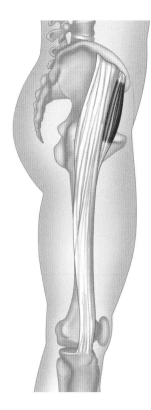

1. The Trochanteric Fan

Hub: Greater trochanter of the femur
Rim: Iliac crest and posterior ischium
Muscles: Tensor fasciae latae (TFL); gluteus medius and minimus; gluteus maximus, superior portion; piriformis (apex); gemellus superior and inferior; obturator internus and externus; quadratus femoris (transition)

The abductor group starts with the TFL, reaching down and back from the ASIS to the upper front aspect of the greater trochanter, as well as reaching down into the thigh and even below the knee via the anterior portion of the ITT. As such, it can help to flex the hip, medially rotate the hip, and, of course, participate in abducting the hip.

Figure 6.14: Tensor fasciae latae and the iliotibial tract.

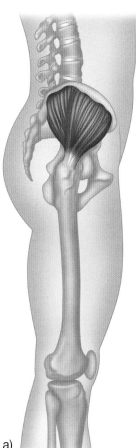

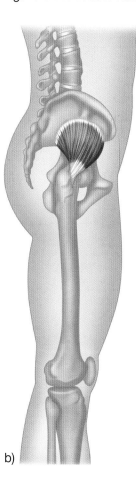

The gluteus medius, and its denser little brother minimus, attach from the whole outside of the flange of the ilium (the gluteal fossa) to the top outside of the greater trochanter. Like the deltoid in the shoulder, they can participate in either medial or lateral rotation depending on which fibers are employed, as well as act together to strongly abduct the leg.

a)

b)

Figure 6.15: a) gluteus medius and b) gluteus minimus.

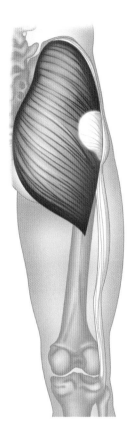

The gluteus maximus is really two muscles, and the upper part (from the hip bone) can be seen as part of this fan, extending the hip and helping in abduction. The lower part (from the sacrum and sacrotuberous ligament) is a hip extensor.

Although we practice abduction when we throw our leg over a horse or a hurdle, these muscles are more often (in every step) called upon to prevent adduction. When we bear weight on one leg, the pelvis would like to tilt toward the unweighted leg, and the abductors prevent that tilt. With the abductors absent – as in polio or cerebral palsy – the weight must be passed fully from one hip to the other with each step, or the person must employ the *Trendelenburg gait*.

Figure 6.16: Gluteus maximus.

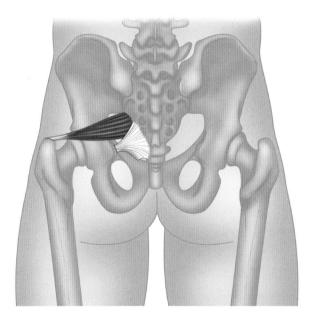

The piriformis is a small but important muscle reaching from the top of the greater trochanter up and back through the greater sciatic foramen (along with the sciatic nerve) to the front of the sacrum. As such it crosses the hip joint and the sacroiliac joint. This makes it 'longer' (not in a physical sense but in a biomechanical sense) than the other muscles of this fan, which all (except TFL and the upper gluteus, which can be seen to cross two joints via the fascial extension of the ITT) cross only the hip joint itself.

Figure 6.17: Piriformis.

Piriformis is thus an important stabilizer of the sacrum and the sacroiliac joint, contracting on cue (we hope) to force close the sacroiliac (SI) joint at the moment of heel strike. Piriformis's role as a lateral rotator is, in our opinion, dwarfed by its role as an adjustable pelvic stabilizer.

This can be easily seen if we think of the two piriformis muscles on either side as part of one complex; they do in fact join fascially across the front of the sacrum. Taken together, these two muscles make the tiny adjustments to the bottom of the sacrum, just below the fulcrum of the SI joint, to accommodate the forces coming from the side-to-side bending of the spine above.

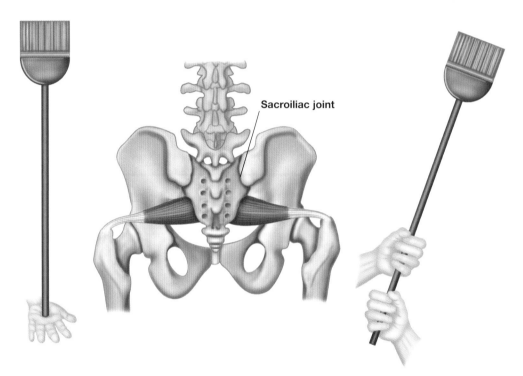

Figure 6.18: The piriformis provides an 'adjustable ligament' to help stabilise the very bottom of the spine. Under sustained strain, the muscles become maladjusted.

Their action could be compared to the tiny adjustments we make with our hand when we are holding a broom upside down in the air. To keep it balanced, we must make constant little adjustments with our palm. If the broom falls beyond our capacity to adjust, then we must grab the broom with one or both fists to keep it from falling. A similar fate befalls the piriformis when the spine is held posturally out of true alignment. No matter what the postural fault, one or both piriformis muscles are likely to bear the burden in a constant state of tension that is hard to resolve unless the problem in the spine above is handled first.

The gemelli lie just superior and inferior to the much larger and more important obturator internus. The gemelli arise essentially from the distal ends of the sacrotuberous and sacrospinous ligaments and may have some role in providing muscular reinforcement to these ligaments. At their distal end, they sometimes blend with the tendon of the obturator internus, such that one can feel one, two, or three tendons here.

The obturator internus is a surprisingly large muscle, because after it turns nearly ninety degrees around the posterior part of the IT, it passes through the lesser sciatic foramen into the pelvic space,

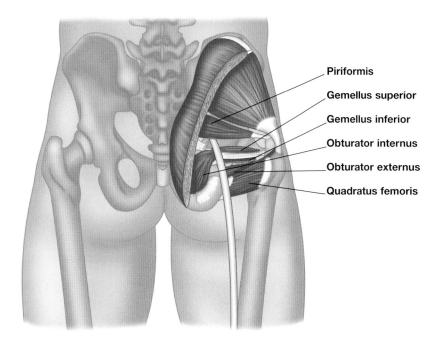

Piriformis

Gemellus superior

Gemellus inferior

Obturator internus

Obturator externus

Quadratus femoris

Figure 6.19: The obturator internus in context with the many surrounding tissues.

spreading to cover the whole obturator foramen – or, in the metaphor of the bones, the whole inside of the lower propeller blade. The lateral tendinous part is accompanied by the two small gemelli muscles above and below it: gemellus superior leading from the sacrospinous ligament, and gemellus inferior leading from the sacrotuberous ligament.

This set of muscles has a powerful lateral rotation force, but also acts to extend the hip and is often overactive in posterior tilt of the pelvis (postural hip extension). These muscles, together with the pelvic floor and sacral ligaments, may also act as 'springs', or a kind of shock absorber for the hip joint.

The obturator externus (barely visible in figure 6.19) is an odd man out in this fan. It is a lateral hip rotator like the others, but due to its originating position on the outside of the lower propeller blade, it accompanies the pubofemoral ligament and acts, unlike any of these others, as a hip flexor, an anterior tilter of the pelvis. This muscle is, in any case, difficult to reach and to treat for the manual therapist.

Quadratus femoris is the transition between the trochanteric fan and the ramic fan, and thus a member of both. Its origin, on the lower posterior side of the IT, marks the end point of the rim of the trochanteric fan, and the beginning of the hub of the ramic fan. Its insertion on the back of the lower part of the greater trochanter marks the beginning of the ramic fan's rim, the linea aspera.

The quadratus femoris itself is a strong stabilizer of the hip, holding the IT to the back of the femur, and helping to maintain the hip extension in which we humans stand.

2. The Ramic Fan

Hub: Ischiopubic ramus
Rim: Medial and lateral linea aspera on the back of the femur
Muscles: Quadratus femoris (transition), adductor minimus, adductor magnus, gracilis (apex), adductor longus, adductor brevis, pectineus (transition)

The ramic fan is more difficult to visualize than either of the others, both because the adductor muscles are usually less familiar to the student, and because the arrangement of the muscles makes the 'rim' of this fan less easily visible. It runs down the outside of the linea aspera and back up the inside, a barely discernible distance between them. If we imagine that instead of opening a fan widely as usual, we left the two ends together and pulled the middle of the fan's rim to its full extent, we would be closer to a parallel to this set of muscle-bone arrangements.

Viewing the thigh from the back, we begin the journey down the lateral side (or the posterior edge, if the leg were turned way out) of the linea aspera with the distal attachment of the quadratus femoris. We can see a set of muscles attaching onto that line. Next down the line is the adductor minimus section of adductor magnus, innervated separately from the obturator nerve.

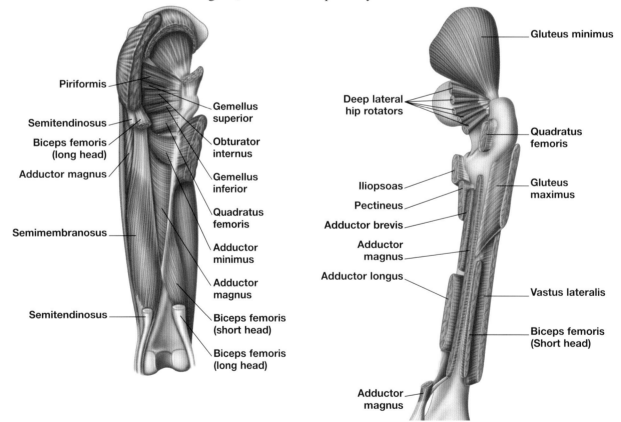

Figure 6.20: The Ramic Fan is easier to see from this angle as a fan folded in on itself. One line descending the posterior aspect of the linea aspera (adductor magnus), then jumping the knee joint with apex muscle of the gracilis (not shown) and then ascending back to the pelvis on the anterior aspect of the linea aspera with the other adductors.

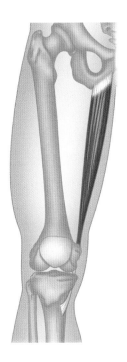

Below that we find the middle of adductor magnus (which we linked to the short head of the biceps femoris in Chapter 5). There is a hiatus separating this section of adductor magnus from the longest part, which goes all the way down to the medial epicondyle of the femur, readily palpable just an inch or so above the medial knee.

The apex of this fan is the gracilis muscle, running from a wide attachment along the bottom of the ischial ramus and crossing both hip and knee to become the middle muscle of the pes anserinus, which we discussed in Chapter 5.

Figure 6.21: Gracilis.

The second half of this fan attaches to the medial or anterior edge of the linea aspera, essentially right beside the adductor magnus, but in a separate fascial plane. The longest of these is, appropriately, adductor longus. This is the large round tendon easily palpable in the groin and usually readily visible if you are seated cross-legged.

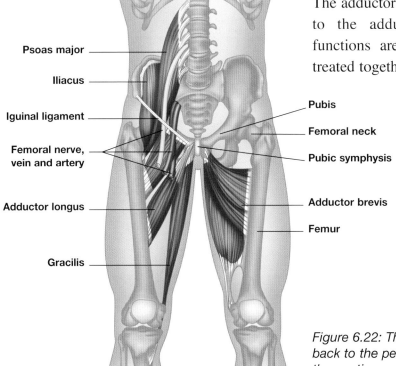

Psoas major

Iliacus

Iguinal ligament

Femoral nerve,
vein and artery

Adductor longus

Gracilis

Pubis

Femoral neck

Pubic symphysis

Adductor brevis

Femur

The adductor brevis lies deep to and superior to the adductor longus, although their functions are so similar that they can be treated together as one entity.

Figure 6.22: The anterior adductors bring us back to the pelvis and to the transition muscle of the pectineus.

The next muscle up on this fan is the transition muscle to the third fan, the pectineus. The distal attachment of pectineus completes the journey up along the medial/anterior portion of the linea aspera to the lesser trochanter, the hub of the final fan. Pectineus is both an adductor and hip flexor. In fact, the back part of the fan (adductor magnus, essentially) is a hip extensor, and all three muscles in the front half of the fan – adductor longus, adductor brevis and pectineus – assist in hip flexion. So this group, or fan, helps to mediate hip flexion and extension, along with the hamstrings and quadriceps we discussed in Chapter 5 and the psoas complex we are about to explore.

Controversy surrounds the role of the adductors in medial and lateral rotation of the hip. While Netter (1989) clearly opts for lateral rotation, Kendall and McCreary (1983) argue for medial rotation. The action may be different depending on the flexion or extension of the hip when the rotation is attempted. But without detailing the arguments (available via 'The Anatomist's Corner' on the Anatomy Trains web site, see appendix), our conclusion is that the adductors play more of a stabilizing role in femoral rotation due to their low moment of rotation relative to the mechanical axis of the femur.

An exception is the pectineus itself when we are talking about the movement of the pelvis on the femur. The pectineus, when shorter on one side, pulls the pubic bone toward that femur; such that we say, when BodyReading the pelvis, 'the pubis points toward the short pectineus'.

3. The Inguinal Fan

Hub: Lesser trochanter of the femur
Rim: Inner edge of the pelvis
Muscles: Pectineus (transition) – links to psoas minor, psoas major (apex), iliacus (links to quadratus lumborum)

Although the third and last fan, which centers around the axis of the lesser trochanter, consists of only three muscles, we will explore two other muscles linked into these three and call the whole thing the *psoas complex*.

Pectineus is our transition muscle – simultaneously an adductor and a deep hip flexor – and is relatively quadrate. The wide proximal attachment on the iliopectineal ridge is matched by a wide distal attachment to the lesser trochanter and the linea aspera below it. Place your fingertips gently into the 'leg pit' – the open space just lateral to the adductor longus tendon – being careful not to press on the femoral artery. Ask the client to bring their knee to the opposite shoulder and feel the pectineus pop into your fingers.

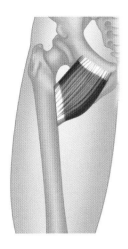

The pectineus links fascially into the psoas minor. This is present in about half your clients as a muscle, according to Travell (1998), but it is present as a fascial strap, according to this author, in nearly everyone. The psoas minor is a thin muscle which may be a highly innervated tension adjuster for the psoas, in the same way that the plantaris is for the Achilles complex or the rectus capitis posterior minor is for the erector spinae complex. In any case, the psoas minor, if present, would flex the lumbar spine and lift the pubic bone to take the pelvis into a posterior tilt.

Figure 6.23: Pectineus.

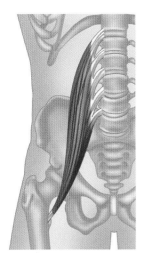

The pectineus–psoas minor complex can be felt and stretched by going into a lunge position with the femur laterally rotated so the knee turns out and your foot is resting more on the big toe side.

The psoas major is the apex muscle in the middle of this fan, running well past the rim of the pelvis to the transverse processes and vertebral bodies of all the lumbars and often the twelfth thoracic vertebrae. It is clearly a strong hip flexor, though its role in hip rotation is less clear (this author suspects it has little role in femoral rotation, see The Anatomist's Corner on the Anatomy Trains web site).

Figure 6.24: Psoas major.

Further, we disagree with the observations of Bogduk (1992) that the psoas has no effect on the lumbar spine. Our own clinical observations suggest that the psoas is essentially a triangular muscle (like the deltoid – look at the psoas in a quadruped to reassure yourself on this point). The fibers that go to the upper lumbars create lumbar flexion and posterior pelvic tilt in the same manner the psoas minor does; the fibers that go to the lower lumbars create lumbar hyperextension, and (through the connection between L5 and the sacrum) ultimately anterior tilt.

Once we understand that the fibers that go to the upper lumbar vertebrae are primarily those in the front and lateral aspect of the psoas major, and that the fibers going to the lower lumbars (the swayback sustainers) are on the inside and posterior portion of the psoas, we can determine a very precise strategy in terms of particular vertebral patterns and positions – as we often see excessive or reverse curvatures in the lumbar vertebrae that make themselves felt in strain patterns above or below that point.

The psoas major is a very rich and sensitive playing field. It joins the upper body and the lower body, the axial to the appendicular skeleton, the inside to the outside, and the back to the front. It is one of the very few muscles with an autonomic plexus within it, and it has intimate relations with the kidneys, intestines and sexuality. Along with the piriformis, it is among the first muscles to go out of balance, and among the last to retain its balance on the way toward integration.

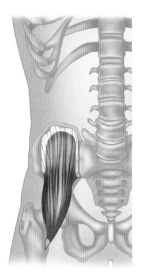

The third muscle of this fan – and the final one that brings us around the ASIS again, where we started at the beginning with the tensor fasciae latae – is the iliacus.

Iliacus has its distal attachment on the lesser trochanter with the psoas major, but passes over the front of the hip joint and under the inguinal ligament a bit lateral to the psoas major to fill in the iliac fossa – or the inside of the upper propeller blade, to use that metaphor one last time. The parallel in the shoulder for the iliacus is the subscapularis, filling in the front of the scapula as the iliacus fills in the front of the ilium.

Figure 6.25: Iliacus.

The proximal attachment of the iliacus is large, running from on or near the ala of the sacrum all along the inner edge of the iliac crest to the ASIS. The iliac fascia, which covers the iliacus and sometimes pulls the psoas major laterally into the iliacus if it is overly tight or bound, is continuous with the quadratus lumborum (QL), which runs to the twelfth rib as well as to the transverse processes of the lumbar vertebrae.

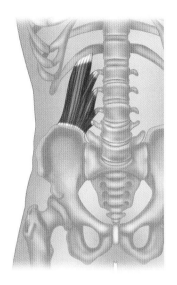

These two muscles form a second complex, running parallel but lateral to the psoas major, passing from the lesser trochanter to the twelfth thoracic vertebra and twelfth rib. This complex can be felt and stretched by going into a lunge position and turning the femur medially, onto the little toe side of the foot. Reaching away from the stretched hip with the ribs on the same side will augment the stretch and bring the complex into sharp relief. Either of the complexes on either side of the psoas major can, in postural compensatory patterns, substitute for a weak or frozen psoas major.

Figure 6.26: Quadratus lumborum.

This completes the cycle of the three fans around the hip joint as we have gone all the way around the propeller from ASIS to ASIS. In practice, of course, these fans work seamlessly during movements to stabilize and mobilize, until something goes wrong that requires one section to work too hard, or prevents it from working at all; such imbalances are readily visible in gait patterns.

Obviously, a similar sweep can be made around the opposite hip joint, but in most people there will be some similarities and some differences between the two in treatment. Sagittal anomalies – an anterior tilt of the pelvis, a flexed lumbar spine, or hyperextended knees – will tend to produce symmetrical compensatory tightness, whereas all rotational patterns, as well as lateral tilts or shifts, will produce asymmetrical patterns. This necessitates good visual and palpatory analysis to develop an effective client-centered strategy.

For instance, one part of the psoas complex may be stabilizing one leg, while another part does the job for the opposite (non-dominant) leg. In pelvic rotational patterns, the right pectineus is often paired with the left piriformis, and vice-versa. While some recurring patterns like these can be identified, the individual peculiarities among these twenty muscles doubled over the two hips provide a variability that requires individual assessment of the entire set. For best results, do visual assessment in standing and walking, as well as a thorough palpatory assessment.

Generally, the transitional myofasciae – pectineus area and quadratus femoris area – will clamp down fascially in significant postural distortion. The pectineus shortens, especially in cases of anterior tilt and medial femoral rotation; the quadratus femoris gets especially fascially thick and short in cases of posterior tilt and lateral femoral rotation.

BodyReading the Pelvis

The pelvis is perhaps the most important area for us to read in relation to its adjacent bones. Most schools of thought give reference to the relationship between the pelvis and the horizontal plane of the ground or the vertical gravitational axis.

Many therapists will have been taught first to measure the angle created between the anterior and posterior superior iliac spines. References differ in suggesting whether this relationship should be level or have a slight angle, and they often indicate that the angle is slightly different between the sexes. Recent research, however, shows these measurements to be quite unreliable, due to the natural variations between people in the shape and size of the bones of the pelvis that affect this angle (Preece et al. 2008). It can still be useful to gain some idea of the orientation and degree of difference, but we have to remember that the angle can vary from anything from zero to twenty-three degrees, when read from a fixed and 'neutral pelvis'. Rather than reading the angle or looking at the relationship of the pelvis to the horizontal floor, we will be better informed about the soft tissue relationships if we look at it in context with the femur.

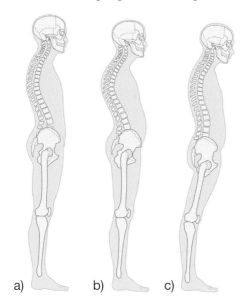

a)   b)   c)

Figure 6.27: Here we see three possible patterns of the skeletal relationships for the femur, pelvis and lumbar spine; (a) neutral pelvis, (b) anterior tilt, (c) anterior shift.

Figure 6.27a shows a pelvis that is neutral both in terms of shift and tilt. But if we look at the soft tissue (figure 6.28), you can see that everything in front and behind the hip joint is in balance.

If we look at figure 6.28a with the trochanteric and inguinal fans added, you can see that all of the muscle fiber crossing in front of the midline of the joint will create hip flexion (anterior tilt) and all the tissue approaching the joint from behind will be extensors (posterior tilt). This gives the fan-like arrangement of these tissues that enables the body to stabilize the femur and pelvis at each phase through the full range of flexion and extension.

Figure 6.28b shows a pelvis that is neutral in shift but anteriorly tilted. This means that the hip joint is in flexion, thereby shortening (or caused by shortened) hip flexors. So if we interpret this from the point of view of the fans, all of the anterior portions will be locked short in both the trochanteric and the ramic. All of the inguinal fan will be locked short (remembering that the psoas major may differ depending on the lumbar pattern). The intermuscular septa will likewise be altered within the adductors – the posterior septum will be drawn up and the anterior one drawn down.

At first sight, figure 6.28c appears to be anteriorly tilted, especially with the degree of hyperlordosis (posterior bend) in the lumbar vertebrae. But once we start to break it down you can see that the pelvis has shifted well in front of the feet, creating an anterior tilt of the femur. We have to read the pelvic tilt in relation to this new angle of the thigh bone and not to the floor. In this case we now see that the pelvis is posteriorly tilted relative to the femurs and therefore it is the posterior elements of the fans, the hip extensors, which may require lengthening.

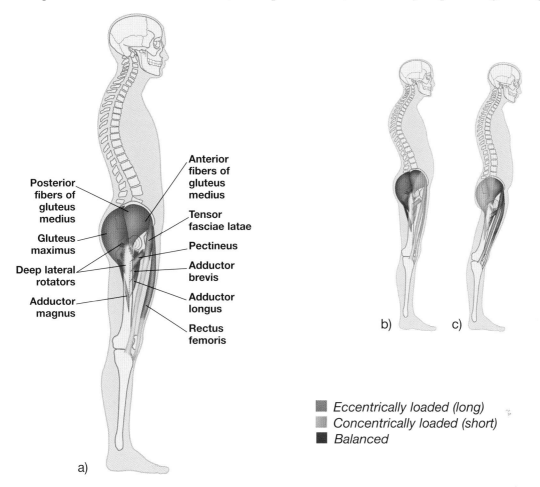

Figure 6.28: By adding the soft tissue onto the forms we can clearly see which areas will be in need of more work.

Between shift and tilt there are nine possible variations of pelvic position:

1 Neutral shift, neutral tilt   2 Anterior shift, neutral tilt   3 Posterior shift, neutral tilt
4 Neutral shift, anterior tilt   5 Anterior shift, anterior tilt   6 Posterior shift, anterior tilt
7 Neutral shift, posterior tilt   8 Anterior shift, posterior tilt   9 Posterior shift, posterior tilt

When working with anterior shifts we need to address the feet, and particularly the heels as seen in Chapter 4, to make sure that the client has enough support posteriorly to come back onto their heels. Then we will also need to address the planes of the fascia, lifting the front and dropping the back.

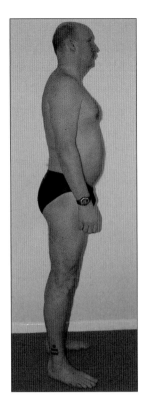

When we look at figure 6.29 with this in mind, then we will see the pelvis as being quite neutral in terms of tilt relative to the femur. The posterior bend of the lumbar vertebrae is created by the posterior tilt of the rib cage, and you can clearly see the length of the abdomen compared to the low back.

Fig 6.29: A client demonstrates an anteriorly shifted pelvis which is neutral in terms of tilt.

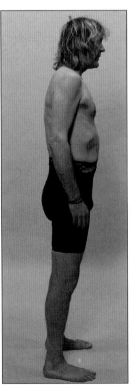

In figure 6.30 we again see an anterior shift and tilt of the femur – and, though more difficult to see, the pelvis appears to be slightly posteriorly tilted when we read it relative to the femur.

Figure 6.30: Here we see the common pattern of a posterior tilt coupled with an anterior shift of the pelvis.

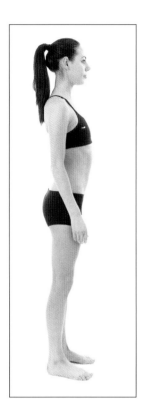

The model in figure 6.31 also demonstrates a slight anterior shift of the pelvis, with the common coupling of a posteriorly tilted rib cage, but on looking at her pelvis it appears slightly anteriorly tilted. In order to lift the compression this pattern creates in her lumbar vertebrae, she compensates by extending her posterior bend of the spine well beyond her upper lumbar vertebrae, possibly as high as T5 or T6.

Figure 6.31: Looking at our model we can see a different pattern in terms of the tilt in the pelvis.

The three fans of the hip are all crossing a ball-and-socket joint capable of movement in all planes. Each of the muscles can then be seen to be involved with a range of patterns depending on the angle at which they cross that joint. For example, when we see lateral tilts of the pelvis, then we need to balance the relationship between the abductors (trochanteric fan) of the low side with the adductors (inguinal fan) of the opposite thigh, as both can be locked short.

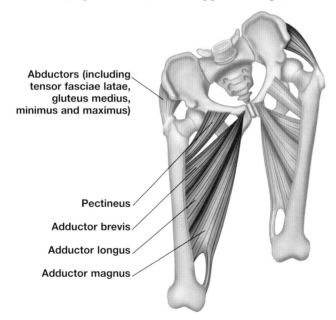

Figure 6.32: In cases of lateral tilts, the abductors will be shortened on the low side, drawing the ilium toward the greater trochanter. This will draw the ischiopubic ramus closer to the opposite, high hip side.

In terms of rotations, the more horizontal a muscle is when it crosses the line of joint action, the more potential it will have to rotate. When the pelvis is pulled to one side, for example, in a right rotation of the pelvis, then the pectineus may be short on the right but the lateral rotators on the left may also be short.

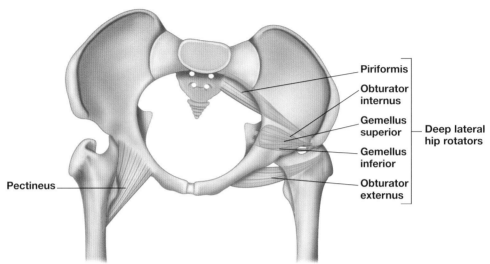

Figure 6.33: When the pelvis rotates to the right the pubic ramus will move closer to the right femur (shortening pectineus) and the left ischial ramus will move closer to the femur on the left (shortening all of the lateral rotators on the left).

The body balances via many of these inter-operating agonist/antagonist relationships that the thorough therapist must watch for, as many are not drawn from the classical anatomy textbooks and so may not always be as obvious as one would expect.

Pelvic Techniques

Clearing the Trochanters (LTL)

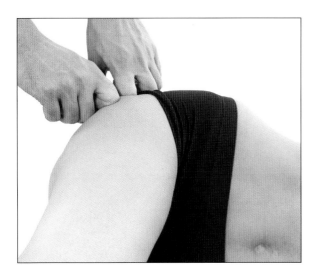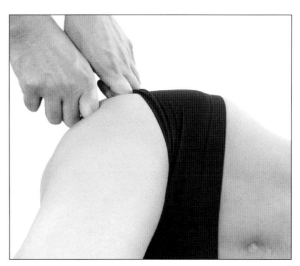

Figure 6.34a & b: Using the knuckles to open the tissue over the greater trochanters with a rolling action from the shoulders and allowing the hands to roll around each other to reduce strain in the arms and wrists.

The tissue over the greater trochanters can often feel as if it has become bound onto the bone and is no longer free to glide independently. Postural issues, especially side tilts of the pelvis, can lead to extra strain on the structures of the lateral hip; and so it can be very relieving, particularly to the underlying trochanteric bursa, to differentiate this tissue.

Position your client in side-lying, with the upper thigh flexed and supported on a bolster, the lower thigh straight. Use the flat surface of the knuckles of both index and middle fingers to spread and open the superficial tissue over the greater trochanter. Start with both fists together and then gently roll them around one another to create the movement, making it an easier and more relaxed contact, rather than pulling the hands apart from the shoulders. The client can assist the opening with a small anterior and posterior tilt of the pelvis while you are working.

Cleaning the Edges of the Ilium (LTL)
The muscle attachments on both the inner and the outer aspect of the iliac crest can quite often become lined with restrictions, knots and nodules in the tissue, often binding the layers together to reduce side-bending and rotation in the trunk.

With the client lying as above, use your fingertips along the superior aspect of the iliac crest to spread the tissue with both sets of fingertips working out from the midline in a neutral pelvis or to get the tissue warmed up. Bring the tissue next to the crest posteriorly from ASIS to PSIS in the case of an anteriorly tilted pelvis, and vice-versa for a posterior tilt.

Above the iliac crest you will be manipulating the abdominal layers. You can gain more specificity by working along the three differing depths for the external and internal obliques and transversus abdominis muscles on the outside of the iliac crest, the top of the crest and the inside of the lip of the crest respectively.

An alternative method for taking the tissue forward or back is to use the flat edge of the ulna. Sitting on the couch behind your client, you can hook the tissue with the forearm closest to the client's body, using your other hand posteriorly to stabilize and support their pelvis. The client

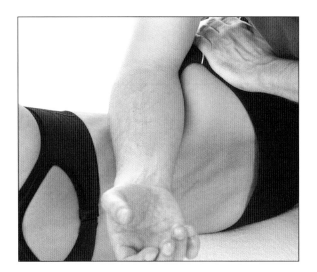

can assist with a small anterior and posterior tilt of the pelvis, or by rotating the rib cage away from the direction you are taking the tissue.

Figure 6.35: Using the ulnar blade to carry the tissue posteriorly.

The ulnar blade is ideal for opening the tissue below the iliac crest, as this tissue tends to be denser and therefore likely to strain your fingers. Knuckles may be a good substitute if you want a slightly more sensitive tool. These tissues – gluteus maximus, gluteus medius and tensor fasciae latae, along with the superior attachments of the fascia lata – can all be spread downward, away from the crest, or moved anteriorly or posteriorly, depending on the client's pattern.

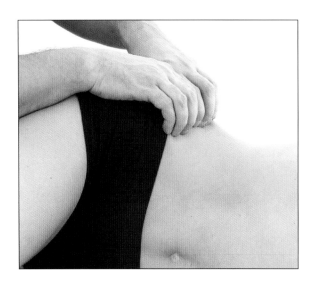
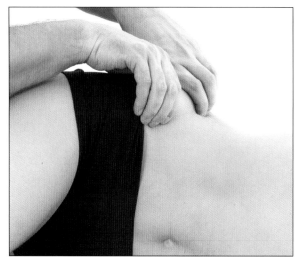

Figure 6.36a & b: Spreading the abdominal attachments, ideal for a neutral pelvis.

All of the above techniques should be accompanied by client movement, most commonly anterior and posterior tilting of their pelvis. This cannot only aid the return of the tissue to a better neutral position but also help re-educate and strengthen many of the weakened muscles around the low back and pelvic complex. It can be particularly beneficial to emphasize the opposite movement to their natural pattern to aid opening their shorter tissue and to break the sensori-motor amnesia cycle in any weak muscles.

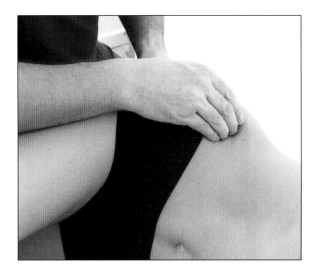

Figure 6.37: Taking the tissue posteriorly for an anteriorly tilted pelvic pattern.

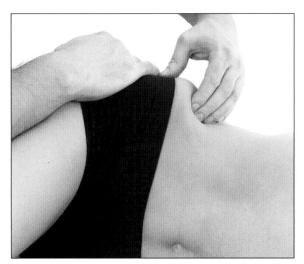

Figure 6.38: Bringing the fascia forward for a posteriorly tilted pelvic pattern.

Opening the Fan (LTL)

From the same position you can use a flat or pointed elbow to work out along the fan of muscles that attach to the greater trochanter. Starting from the greater trochanter you can work up and forward to the ASIS along the TFL and then fan gradually back toward the PSIS and the upper portion of the gluteus maximus. Along the way you will have worked on the anterior and posterior (flexor and extensor) portions of the gluteus medius, but you may wish to avoid the upper portion of the ITT, the thick fascial line around the midline.

The work can be done in simple lines or combined with hip flexion and extension by having the client glide their knee back and forth along the bolster, as you can either pin and stretch in each section or glide along the fibers in the opposite direction.

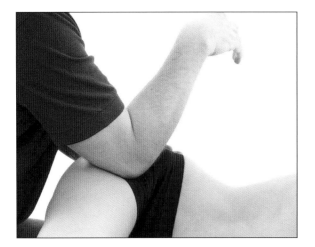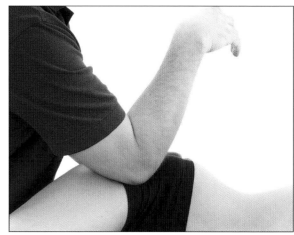

Figure 6.39a & b: Work the anterior portion of the trochanteric fan as the client extends their hip by gliding their knee down along the bolster. Emphasis is placed on the 'locked short' tissues, i.e. everything in front of the midline in an anterior tilted pattern, and vice-versa for a posterior tilt.

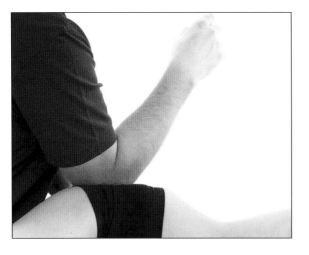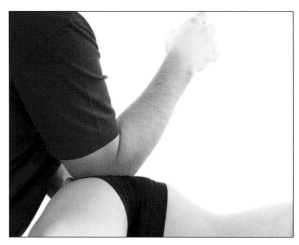

Figure 6.40a & b: Working with the posterior portion of the fan (the extensors) as the client flexes their hip, gliding their thigh along the bolster.

Gluteus Minimus (LTL)

As gluteus minimus is much deeper, underlying gluteus medius, it requires a slightly different working position. The client's thigh must be passively abducted in order to shorten and relax the overlying medius and superficial fascia lata tissue. Either support the client's foot on your own hip, holding their knee in your lower hand, or slide your lower arm under their knee, with their leg resting on your forearm and their inner knee in your hand.

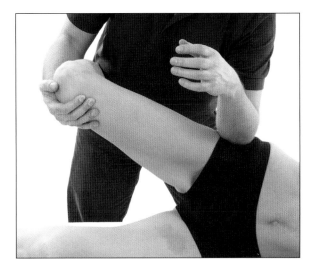 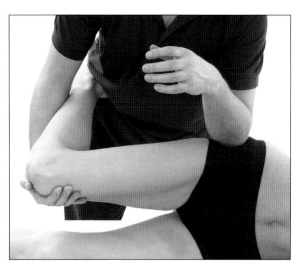

Figure 6.41a & b: Passively abduct the thigh to keep the superficial abductors relaxed, and using a sensitive elbow sink through them to engage the deeper gluteus minimus, and then slowly adduct the thigh back to neutral. Because it lies mostly along the midline it will be more involved with lateral tilts of the pelvis rather than anterior/posterior issues.

Sink your elbow attentively into the deeper tissue around the lateral midline superior to the greater trochanter. Have your client engage their adductors by pushing into your supporting arm or hand to help remove some of the protective tension through reciprocal inhibition. This is a very sensitive and untouched area for most clients, so sometimes you must be patient and try different images to obtain their relaxed consent. Once you have engaged the deeper myofascia and hooked toward the ilium, you can then slowly lower the knee back to the table as you maintain the connection into the gluteus minimus, creating a unique stretch on its tissue.

Working with the Iliotibial Tract (LTL)

Now that you have released the tissues which determine much of the tension on the often notoriously tight iliotibial tract (ITT), it should be eased and a little more susceptible to manipulation. Working from the hip to the knee, you can use your ulna or fingers (if strong enough for such a long stroke). Your fist, fingers or ulna can be used if working from the knee to the hip. Generally the tissue needs to be spread away from the lateral midline on the underlying vastus lateralis, but may be worked superiorly or inferiorly at the same time, depending on the client's pattern.

Using your ulna like the bow of a violin, you can focus on any aspect of the lateral thigh more in need of work, whether it be the anterior or posterior portion of the ITT. These can also be taken in different directions determined by the pelvic position of the client; work up the front and down the back to help correct an anterior pelvis, and the opposite direction for one with a posterior tendency.

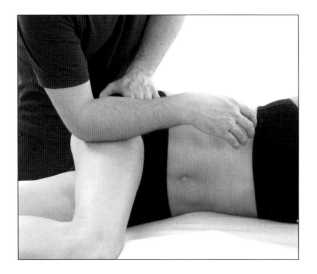 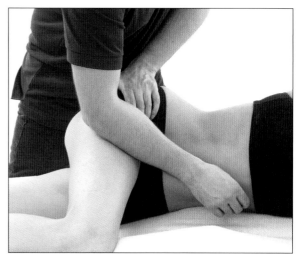

Fig 6.42a & b: Use your ulna to address different aspects of the ITT, which may need to be brought superiorly or inferiorly along its anterior or posterior aspects, depending on the client's pelvic tilt.

The technique is shown working inferiorly, but could equally be traveling up the outside of the thigh if you were to stand on the opposite side of the table. Other possibilities would be to use the fist, or fingers.

Piriformis

Piriformis is a crucial muscle in pelvic positioning and balance. As the apex muscle of the trochanteric fan it crosses two joints, the hip and the sacroiliac joint. As it crosses the back of the hip joint it will be shortened in a posterior tilt of the pelvis similarly on both sides. In cases of lateral tilts of the pelvis, sacrum or lower spine and pelvic rotations, then you will need to create more balance between the piriformis on either side of the body.

You can find piriformis by palpating your client's PSIS and coccyx and drawing a line from halfway between those points to the greater trochanter. The muscle runs from the anterior surface of the sacrum down and out to the top of the femur, so by strumming in a superolateral/inferomedial direction in the middle of this line you should feel the deep and small 'speed bump' of the muscle belly. Spending time waiting for the muscle to ease and sinking gradually deeper into its layers can be useful prior to locking into it by either dropping your shoulder proximally to give an outward stretch to the proximal fibers or pushing medially to isolate the stretch in the distal portion.

Both of these methods should be combined with lateral rotation of the femur by the client. The piriformis is small and lies under the thick gluteus maximus, so it cannot always be felt clearly. But if you follow the directions above, you will be working with the piriformis, whether you can feel its tendon distinctly or not.

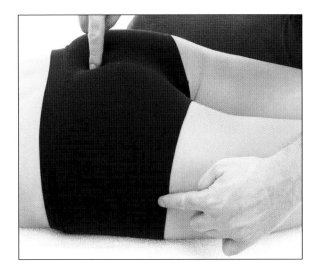 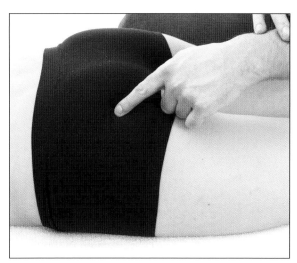

Figure 6.43a & b: Finding the piriformis by locating the halfway point along the center of the sacrum and then locating the point halfway between it and the greater trochanter.

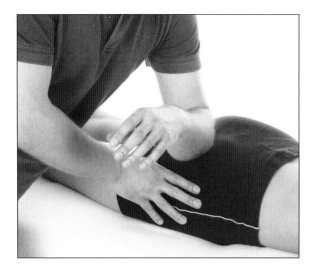 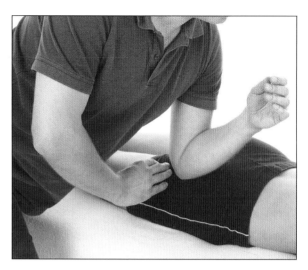

Figure 6.44a & b: Using your elbow, sink through the overlying gluteals and lock into the tissue of the piriformis. A fascial stretch can be achieved by then taking your shoulder across the midline of the body to create a lateral stretch on the tissue. This could be combined with having the client medially rotate their thigh.

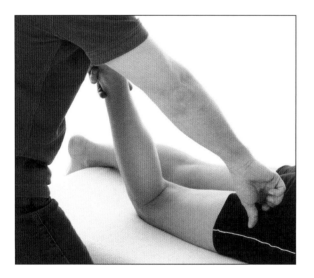 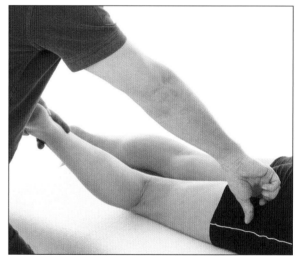

Figure 6.45a & b: Using your knuckles, engage the piriformis, and then actively or passively medially rotate the thigh to open the tissue. In this position the lock is angled toward the midline of the body and therefore isolates the distal portion of the piriformis.

Obturator Internus (DFL)

The lateral part of obturator internus and the gemelli muscles can be approached in a similar manner, just inferior to the piriformis and superior to the gluteal fold. In some clients, there will be two or three distinctly palpable tendons, but in many these three will feel like on large tendon. Bring these tissues down in the case of an anteriorly tilted pelvis; work them laterally in the case of a posteriorly tilted pelvis.

With courage and permission, you can get valuable work done on the belly of the obturator internus. With your client side-lying, locate the ischial tuberosity on their lower side. Then use the sacrotuberous ligament as your guide, by keeping the side of your finger in contact with it as you swim anteriorly and superiorly (in the direction of the navel) to reach past the ischium to come into contact with the obturator internus muscle.

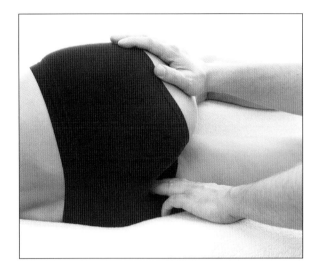

Figure 6.46: Explain to your client exactly where you are going to work and why, before locating the obturator internus by mindfully sinking medially and inferiorly to the sacrotuberous ligament.

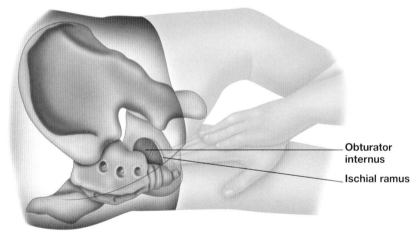

Obturator internus

Ischial ramus

Figure 6.47: Here we can see more clearly the fingertips gliding along the inside of the ischial ramus and following the to contact the obturator internus. The three dimensions of the pelvis are difficult to grasp from a diagram and this technique may be best learnt under supervision for the novice practitioner.

As you engage the tissue, ask your client to slowly rotate their leg medially to release it. This technique is especially important for those with a posteriorly tilted pelvis, or for those with what the Americans call 'tight-ass syndrome'. Remember that you are near the anal verge and affecting the pelvic floor by working in this area. It is best to practice this technique initially with a friendly colleague, approaching it in practice with care, communicating clearly where you will be and why you will be working in this area.

Quadratus Femoris

Find the quadratus femoris belly by coming out and slightly up from the lower edge of the ischial tuberosity; it will feel like a softer rounded speed bump. Contact into it, drawing the tissue proximally or distally, and ask your client to slowly roll their leg medially.

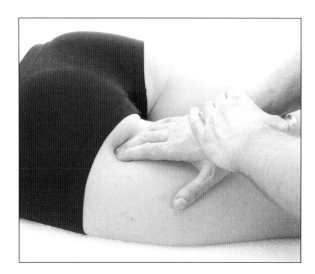 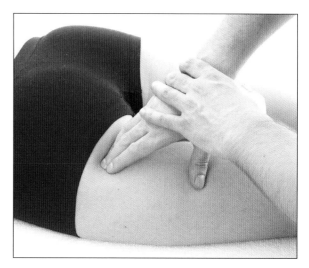

Figure 6.48a & b: Find the quadratus femoris tissue by first locating the ischial tuberosity and then sinking into the tissue laterally and slightly superiorly to it. Engage the tissue laterally (as shown) or medially, as the client medially rotates their thigh.

Adductors – The Ramic Fan (DFL)

Many practitioners of bodywork spend little time with the adductors. They are tucked away on the inside of the thigh, an intimate area. They are often tender and tight, and even the overlying skin seems to be thinner and less robust than that of the anterior thigh. So it is little wonder that this is often one of the first areas to be omitted when time is short. Few clients may request you to work in this area but, with conscientious assessment and sensitive technique, many will later thank you if you do.

We said above that the adductors are involved with nearly all of the actions of the thigh except abduction. The adductor group is also particularly active in pelvic stabilization, and so are often bound up, tight and knotted. Additionally, it is not uncommon for this area to be emotionally 'loaded', so work slowly and with compassion.

To get a sense of the territory, we use a simple exercise. With the client in side-lying, and using the same side hand as that of the client's thigh, place the flat of your hand approximately mid-thigh, with your fingers slightly spread. Allowing for variations in width of thigh and span of hand, your thumb should be roughly on top of the sartorius. The adductor longus will be under your index finger, and gracilis under the middle finger. Adductor magnus is deep to the ring finger. Your spread little finger will then be over the rounded bellies of the medial hamstrings.

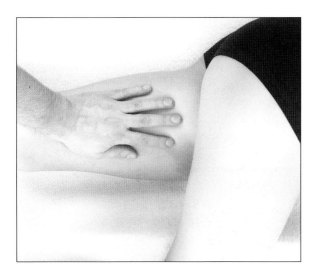

Figure 6.49: Showing the fingers spread to orientate to the adductors. The thumb should feel a slight groove deep to the slender sartorius (the position of the anterior septum). The index finger will feel the rounded bump of the adductor longus, middle finger will be over the gracilis and your ring finger will be on the adductor magnus. The little finger should be able to sink between the hamstrings and the adductor magnus (the posterior septum).

Working on the lower thigh with your client in side-lying, use your soft fists to sink into and simply work the adductor tissue away from the midline. You can use the same rolling action of your fists around each other, or cross your arms to allow your weight to do the work.

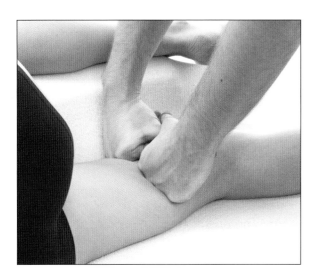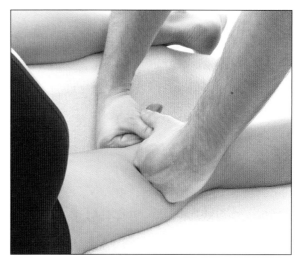

Figure 6.50a & b: Spreading the adductor tissue by sinking into them and slowly rolling your fists to open the tissue. An alternative is to cross your hands and simply drop your bodyweight into the movement to create the stretch.

Your aim for this movement is primarily to open the septa between the quadriceps and the adductors anteriorly and the adductors and the hamstrings posteriorly. But it can also act as a general introduction to the adductors, giving you the opportunity to assess where they may need more attention.

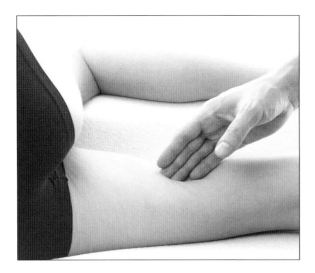 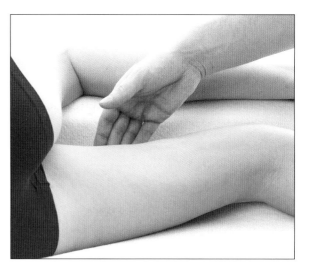

Figure 6.51a & b: Working the posterior and anterior septa using fingertips. The direction can change depending on the pelvic pattern.

The septa can then be opened with a sharper tool such as your fingertips, or perhaps even knuckles in the football player's thigh. The septa can be lifted or dropped, depending on the pattern of pelvic tilt (i.e. up the anterior septum and down the posterior for an anteriorly tilted pelvis, or vice-versa for a posteriorly tilted pelvis).

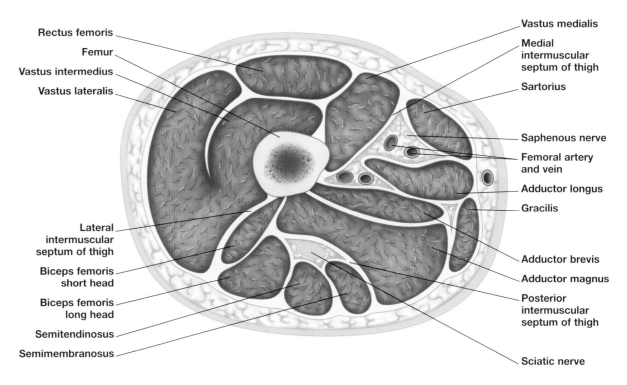

Figure 6.52: The septa divide the various muscle groups of the thigh, but also often act as channels for the passage of the neurovascular bundles.

Take care when working with the anterior septum underlying the sartorius, as it contains the femoral neurovascular bundle. Rather than directing your force straight into the thigh, angle it slightly against either wall to avoid occluding or impinging any of these vessels. Nerve tingling in the client or the feeling that you are pressing on something that is pulsing underneath you (both rare) would be reason to retreat and try a different angle.

Leg Lengthening

The tissue on the inside of the '7' of the femur (in and around the lesser trochanter) can often become restricted, affecting hip extension and abduction. By dropping soft fingertips into the space between the gracilis and the adductor magnus, you can gain access into the space near the lesser trochanter. Ask your client to then reach down the table away from the hip with their heel, as you draw the tissue on the inside of the hip joint inferiorly by curling your fingers (having

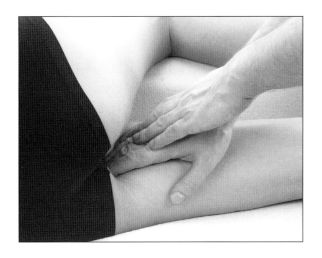

them supported with the digits of the upper hand can help soften the contact fingers and give them more strength). Although deep work in this area can be breathtaking at first, the rewards in terms of easy walking or a lengthened leg are worth the time and effort to reach mutual accommodation in getting down near the inner aspect of the femur.

Figure 6.53: Sink your fingers into the hollow between the adductor magnus and the gracilis just inferior to the ischial ramus and ease the tissue toward the foot as it reaches out along the table.

Pelvic Floor (DFL)

With your client in side-lying and the upper thigh flexed and bolstered, use the sacrotuberous ligament of the upper hip to guide your fingers toward the navel until you contact the pelvic floor with your fingertips. When you feel it, you can then use the contact for educating the client. The direct feedback can be used as a guide to clients who have difficulty in isolating or controlling their pelvic floor muscles and often need to develop more tone. If you find that it is already quite high and toned, then hook your fingers slightly to draw the tissue downward. Remember to work with full awareness and permission of your client if you are attempting this move.

A variation of this move can be done with the client sitting on the table with feet on the floor. Have them lift one 'cheek' and from the side slide your fingers (carefully – do not go too far!), so that your fingertips are just hooked around the ischial tuberosity. Exert a gentle lateral pressure, as if to pull the IT toward you, while the client slowly and gently rocks between an anterior and posterior tilt for thirty seconds or more. When you take your hand out, have the client sit on both ITs before you do the other side. Just this simple technique will often produce a very palpable difference for the client in how the pelvis is supported.

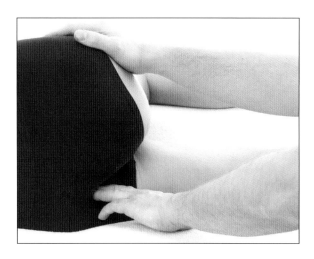

Figure 6.54: Using the sacrotuberous ligament as your guide, glide along the medial surface of the obturator internus until your fingertips come against a soft barrier.

Pectineus (DFL)

With your client lying supine, knees bent up, come in over the thigh and use the long round tendon of the adductor longus as a guide for the ring finger of your inner hand to slide your palm along the inside of the thigh toward the fold at the top of the inner anterior thigh, right beside the the pubic bone, being careful not to overstretch the skin.

Check that you are engaged into the pectineus tissue by asking your client to lift their thigh toward their opposite shoulder while you give resistance with your forearm, enhancing the contraction of the muscle and giving your fingertips a positive 'bounce' to ensure your accuracy.

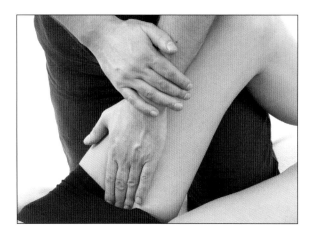 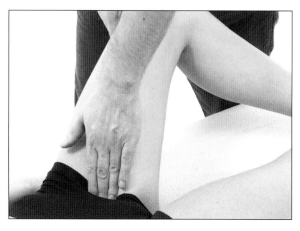

Figure 6.55a & b: Use the rounded tendon of the adductor longus as your guide (if you can't find it ask the client to adduct their thigh against your hand, taking it toward their opposite shoulder, and it should pop up). Make sure you are not pressing on the pulse of the femoral artery, and then, after checking that you are engaged in the myofascia of the pectineus, slowly abduct the thigh. You can use your non-working hand to guide the knee down. Even using reciprocal inhibition by asking the client to push out against it can help reduce any resistance.

To challenge the distal portion of the pectineus, hook toward the pelvis as the client drops their knee outward (as above). To isolate the stretch on the proximal portion, hook toward the femur and ask your client to push into their standing foot and slowly turn their pelvis and trunk as if to look over their opposite shoulder.

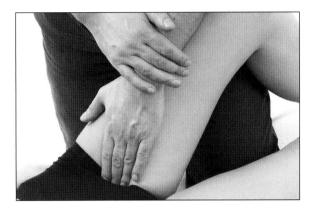
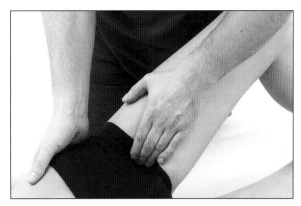

Figure 6.56a & b: With your fingers in the same starting position as above, hook the tissue laterally. Then ask your client to push into their foot to turn their body (particularly the pelvis) as if they are trying to look over their opposite shoulder. This technique takes the proximal attachment (along the pubic ramus) away from the femoral attachment and so isolates a different portion of the tissue, as well as having a stronger movement re-education element.

Iliacus (DFL)

Bring a little of the loose skin from the belly laterally to the ASIS as this will allow your fingers to drop into the iliac fossa just medial and slightly superior (to avoid the inguinal ligament) to the boney landmark without overstretching the skin. The iliacus will be just under your fingerpads; the iliac fascia is ahead of your fingertips and the psoas major muscle, if you are deep enough, will be against your fingernails. If your way is impeded into the valley between the iliacus and the psoas, open the iliac fascia by gently swimming or prizing your way through it, to allow the iliacus and psoas major to work separately.

By connecting, into the iliacus and its fascia on the inside of the pelvic bowl, you can put tension into the tissue of the iliacus by hooking it superiorly and asking your client to slowly glide their heel along the table to straighten their leg. Finally, get them to reach down and out with their heel, to further challenge and open the tissue away from your fingertips.

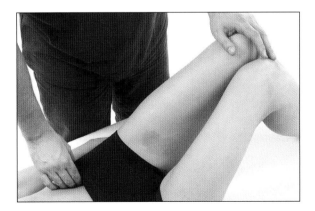
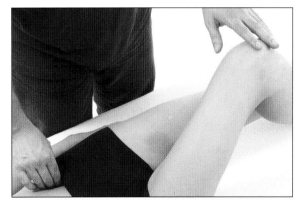

Figure 6.57a & b: With the client's knees flexed, sink slowly inside the iliac fossa and engage the iliac fascia superiorly to resist the lengthening as the client glides their heel along the table to straighten the leg.

To add a further level of sophistication, you can also train your client to engage their abdominals lightly (too much tension will push you out or create pain and discomfort) to maintain a neutral tilt of their pelvis as they lengthen their leg away. This can help bring awareness, control and tone to otherwise weakened muscles, to enhance the long-term effects of your work.

Psoas (DFL)

This deep and structurally important muscle benefits from respect in both approach and treatment. Position your client supine with their knees bent, feet flat on the table, heels close to the buttocks.

By sinking into the same area as for the iliacus, you can keep traveling medially, following the contour of the iliac fossa to guide your way to the lateral fibers of the psoas major. Approaching the psoas major from this angle allows you the opportunity to assess the relative positions and relationship of the psoas major and the iliacus, as they can often become bound together by the iliac fascia, as discussed in the previous section. The psoas major can migrate slightly laterally when that happens.

You may need to spend some time 'teasing' the psoas major free from the iliacus if the two have become bound together. The psoas major itself can be worked according to the client's pelvic pattern; if anteriorly tilted, focus on the medial fibers, or on the lateral fibers if the pelvis is posteriorly tilted or the client is showing a flatback pattern.

You will contact the lateral fibers first when approaching the psoas major from the side. If you need to get to the medial fibers, keep your fingers in contact with the muscle, gliding or walking them over the muscle belly to reach the shorter medial portion. By staying in contact with the myofascia of the psoas major, you will hopefully ease any of the sensitive viscera out of the way before pressing onto and stretching the tissue.

Be careful when working in this area, and stay below the level of the navel. Ask the client to warn you if they feel any gas-like or sharp searing pain, or if they need to cough, sneeze or laugh (refrain from telling any jokes as you work this area!). All of these will require you to withdraw and either sink into a slightly different section or allow the discomfort to settle.

Engage either section of the psoas major depending on the pattern, hooking the tissue superiorly, and then ask your client to slowly lengthen their leg away, sliding their heel along the table and finally reaching it away.

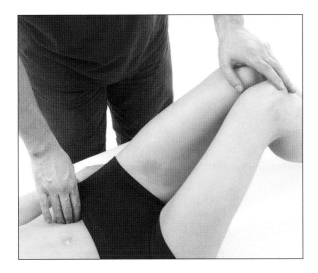
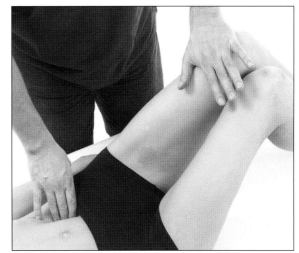
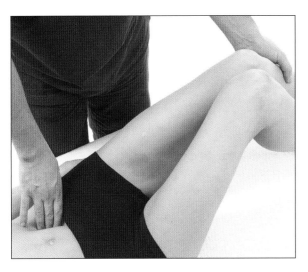
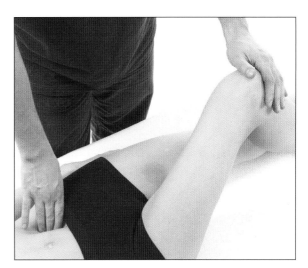

Figure 6.58a, b, c & d: Gently, sink into the iliac fossa using your 'head' hand, letting gravity and your bodyweight do as much of the work as possible. Use the shape of the iliac fossa to guide you deep and then medial. To check for the location of the psoas major, ask the client to lift their foot off the table to push their knee into your resisting hand, which increases the contraction of the muscle under your palpating hand. Engage into whichever aspect of psoas major is required (medial or lateral) and have the client slowly glide their foot down along the table to lengthen.

Be sure that you finish up with a simple, bilateral balancing move, when working the two psoas major muscles differently (as you would in a lumbar side-bending or spinal rotoscoliosis pattern). With the client still supine with knees up, engage the psoas major gently and equally on both sides, and have the client rock the pelvis slowly on the table through several anterior and posterior tilts. Even if one psoas major is very much shorter than the other and has engaged all of your attention up to now, because the psoas major is such a physiologically and neurologically rich muscle, you will leave your client in a better place if you finish your work with a bilateral balancing move. Irritable Bowel Syndrome or other inflammations of the intestine constitute a contraindication for this work, or at the very least a warning to move very slowly and sensitively.

The Abdomen, Thorax, and Breathing

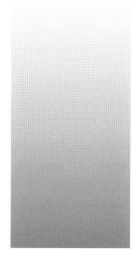

The Abdomen and Ribs: Support for the Ventral Cavity

Having worked our way up the legs, we come to a natural functional division between the legs and torso, and we now follow that traditional separation, but with one word of caution. The legs are not only the biomechanical foundation for the spine; the two are interlinked viscerally and fascially in many ways.

The fascia lata of the Lateral Line, although it attaches to the iliac crest, is a continuous fabric with the abdominal fasciae of the lateral external and internal obliques. The hamstrings, via the sacrotuberous ligament, are continuous with the erector spinae, which we will discuss in Chapter 8. Finally, the core tissues of the Deep Front Line connect the septum between the hamstrings and adductors to the pelvic floor and anterior sacrum posteriorly, and run through the 'leg pit' into the abdominal cavity anteriorly with the psoas major and iliacus. Thus, the 'natural' separation between legs and trunk is a false one, with the viscera extending themselves into the legs via the nerves and vessels, and the legs themselves originating from behind the organs at the twelfth rib and lumbar vertebrae.

That said, the term 'ventral cavity' is a useful one. It comprises the smaller cavities at the superior end – oral, nasal, pharyngeal – and the larger thoracic, abdominal, and pelvic, which we will now explore from the bottom up.

The Abdominal Balloon

Although the division between the abdominal – much of what is below the diaphragm – and the pelvic – the organs of the true deep pelvis that lie below the peritoneum – is useful surgically, in muscular terms these two cavities can be considered together. They are bounded above by the respiratory diaphragm, and below by the pelvic floor or pelvic diaphragm. Achieving a balanced reciprocity between these two structures is essential to long-term human biomechanical health.

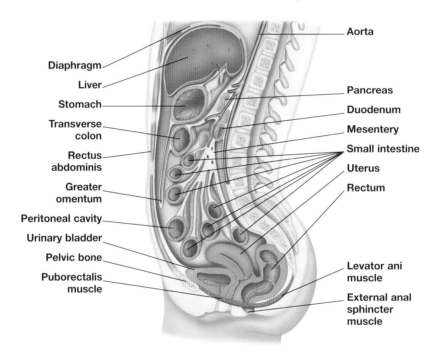

Figure 7.1: The abdomino-pelvic organs are held between the resilient respiratory diaphragm above and the pelvic floor below.

Getting to that balance is somewhat a function of the healthy tone and movement of these two muscles – diaphragm and levator ani – but relies even more on the balance among the elements in the tube of myofasciae that lie between them, holding in the organs and holding up the trunk. These consist principally of the 'Union Jack' of abdominal muscles along the front and sides: rectus abdominis, transversus abdominis and the external and internal abdominal obliques. Along the back wall lie the psoas major and quadratus lumborum, as well as the spine itself. In the pelvis, we also have smaller exposure of the piriformis and obturator internus near the pelvic floor.

Since we have dealt with these latter muscles in Chapter 6, we will concentrate on the four large sheets of myofascia known as the *abdominal muscles* and some interesting fascial tracks within them, before moving on to the movements of the diaphragm and the ribs.

The Union Jack of Abdominal Muscles

Sticking with the Union Jack image for a minute, the cross of St. Andrew, looking like an 'X', consists of the combined efforts of the contralateral external and internal oblique muscles, working in tandem from the ribs across the center line to the opposite hip. That means that these muscle complexes must work through the rectus fascia and the linea alba in the center.

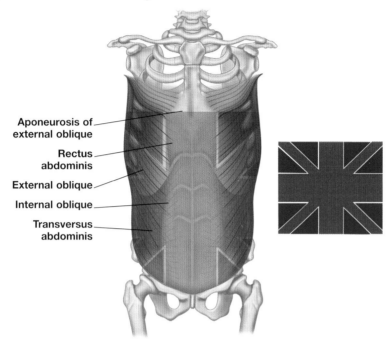

Aponeurosis of external oblique

Rectus abdominis

External oblique

Internal oblique

Transversus abdominis

Figure 7.2: The four bilateral muscles of the abdomen basically resemble a Union Jack, with the obliques forming an 'X', and the rectus abdominis and transversus abdominis forming a cross.

These muscles thus provide stability between the ribs and the pelvis when considered in isometric contraction (as in country dancing). But they can also provide for minor adjustments in the spiraling between ribs and pelvis. This includes alternating a slight shortening of one leg of the 'X' and then the other, as in walking. Or it can be a wild, strong and coordinated shortening of one side over the other, as in African dance or a javelin throw.

These muscles are a combination of square sheets of muscle – usually employed for stability – and triangular muscles – usually employed for a wide range of control. The above paragraph illustrates the need for both in this area. Many times, as in using the shoulders for digging, lifting weights, or most Western dancing, we want to stabilize the trunk on the pelvis in a solid, pressurized position.

The combination of the lumbar and lower thoracic joints, however, amounts to a ball-and-socket joint between the pelvis and the ribs, allowing for flexion, extension, side-bending, rotation and circumduction. These four muscles of the abdominal 'X' can therefore be equally useful in facilitating belly dancing, or giving more leverage to any kind of throw.

These muscles are more complex than the 'X' idea allows. The external oblique, for instance, ties the lower ribs and subcostal cartilage not only to the opposite ASIS (by way of the contralateral internal oblique), but also directly into the ipsilateral pubic bone. Although this connection is strong, it lies right beside a weak place in the abdominal wall, where in men the spermatic cord exits the abdomen on its way to the testicles. Women likewise have an exit here, but only for the round ligament, so they are less likely to produce an inguinal hernia when they increase intra-abdominal strain. While the 'X' we have been describing can best be seen as part of the Spiral Line, this connection to the pubic bone crosses over to the adductors on the opposite side, stabilizing the ribs to the opposite femur. That makes part of this muscle a track in the Front Functional Line.

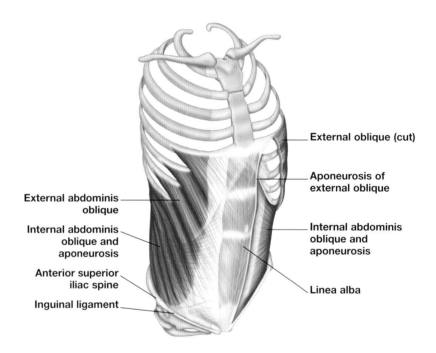

Figure 7.3: The external oblique does not only link with the internal oblique on the other side to connect the ribs to the opposite pelvis (Spiral Line). It also links the ribs to the pubic bone (Front Functional Line) and the ipsilateral iliac crest (Lateral Line).

Looking to the most lateral part of this muscle, we can see that it passes from the posterior lower ribs to the ASIS on the same side. This section has more leverage in side-bending, though it still has some rotational component, but in any case falls more into the territory of the Lateral Line.

The internal oblique is likewise sheet-like but also triangular, reaching up toward the opposite ribs as part of the 'X'. It reaches across to the opposite side of the ASIS to help the transversus abdominus reinforce the lower abdominal wall, and even down along the inguinal ligament toward the pubic bone.

The complementary cross of St. George (like the Red Cross or a plus sign) is formed by the combination of the rectus abdominis running vertically and the transversus abdominis, whose fibers run horizontally, like a large belt around the soft belly. Transversus abdominis is accorded a large role in stabilizing the low back and (along with the sacral multifidi) the sacroiliac joint. The action of the muscle is to squeeze the abdominal contents and create pressure stability in this way – you cannot move a piano without it.

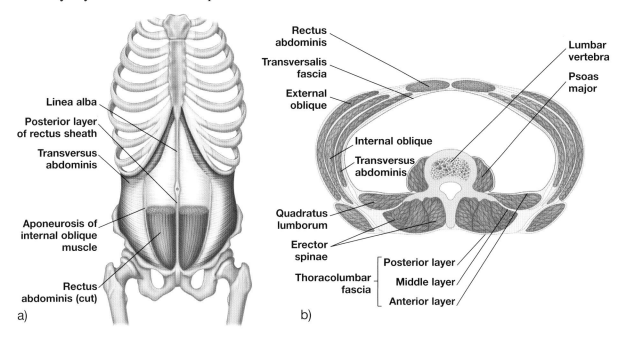

Figure 7.4a & b: a) The transversus abdominis is one of very few muscles whose fibers run horizontally, circumferentially around the body, b) the thoracolumbar fascia around the erector spinae and multifidus completes the transversus 'belt' around our waist, enclosing the quadratus lumborum and psoas major in with the organs.

Research has shown the neurological connection between the transversus abdominis and the pelvic floor. They often co-contract, providing strong stability to the abdomino-pelvic balloon when they work properly, or contributing to urinary incontinence and low back instability when they do not. There are, of course, two transversus abdominis muscles – one left, one right – and they act generally at the deepest level of abdominal fascia, just outside the organic peritoneum, across the linea alba from transverse process to transverse process.

The rectus abdominis is the most widely known of these muscles, being mostly on the outside (though we will dispute this fascially in a minute) and having those wonderful tendinous inscriptions that distinguish a cut 'six-pack' from the beer belly of Joe Six-Pack. These inscriptions essentially turn the rectus abdominis into four muscles on each side. This is a necessity, since the muscle must span such a long way from pubis to sternum without any supporting bone underneath. The inscriptions therefore add strength to our soft underbelly that might otherwise rip in vigorous exercise or reaching.

The rectus abdominis is of course active in trunk flexion, bringing the front of the rib cage closer to the pubic bone in the classic sit-up or crunch, acting across the many costal, lumbar and even sacroiliac joints as it does so. It is also active as a stabilizing muscle like the other abdominals (and like the obliques it is a combination square and triangular muscle). The rectus abdominis further acts as a restraint to hyperextension in the lumbar vertebrae.

Fascial Sheaths in the Abdomen

The rectus abdominis is the most superficial muscle of the belly. Anywhere you stick a pin into the front of the belly, the rectus abdominis would be the first muscle you meet. Fascially, however, it is a different story. Up at the superior attachment at the fifth rib, it is indeed the most superficial muscle. A few centimeters below the ribs, however, the fascia of the external oblique covers the rectus abdominis, so that, fascially speaking, it is now deeper than the external oblique. A bit below that, the fascial extension of the internal oblique covers the rectus abdominis. At the arcuate line, about the level of the *hara* a few centimeters below the navel, it dives behind the transversus fascia to become the deepest muscle of the abdomen by the time it reaches the pubic bone. This provides a connection between the rectus abdominis and the pelvic floor – very useful in considering postpartum problems.

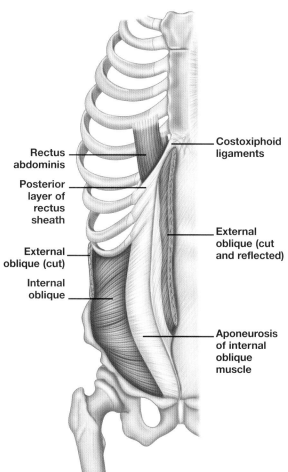

Rectus abdominis

Posterior layer of rectus sheath

External oblique (cut)

Internal oblique

Costoxiphoid ligaments

External oblique (cut and reflected)

Aponeurosis of internal oblique muscle

Figure 7.5: The rectus abdominis may be the most superficial muscle, but in terms of the fascial planes, it moves from being the most superficial at the top to being the deepest – below both obliques and the transversus abdominis – by the time it reaches the pubic bone.

Both the rectus abdominis and the transversus abdominis are essential actors in the two 'belts' we can see in the abdominal balloon. The transversus abdominis muscles, running from transverse process to transverse process via the linea alba in the front, comprise most of the horizontal belt. This is completed by the fascia running around the erector spinae – the superficial and deep laminae of the lumbar fascia – to meet at the spinous processes.

The vertical belt starts with the rectus abdominis, goes up over the top with the central part of the diaphragm to the crura, and continues down the anterior longitudinal ligament to the pelvic floor. The pubococcygeus crosses the bottom of the balloon and this belt, which then meets up with the fascia behind the rectus abdominis once again at the pubic bone. Getting the proper balance around these two belts ensures proper stability and a good foundation for the rib cage and head above.

The Parachute Strings

We must consider one more set of solely fascial structures before we leave this outline of the abdominal mechanics – the four cords of the *parachute*. In this image, we modify the idea of the abdominal balloon to see the diaphragm as a parachute, and the pelvis as the basket underneath the parachute.

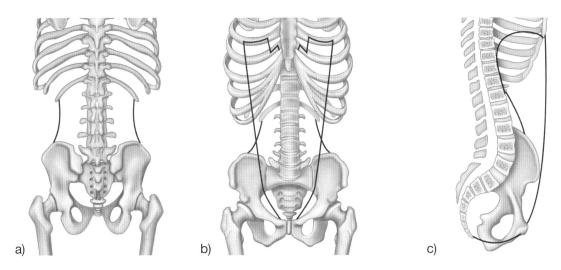

a)   b)   c)

Figure 7.6a, b & c: The fascial connections of the abdomen; a) The corresponding lines in back are known as the lateral raphes. They form a short, strong fascial link between the lower ribs and the posterior iliac crest, b) just outside the rectus abdominis is a place where the various fascial planes of the belly 'seal' together, providing a strong fascial strip between the pubes and the seventh rib, tying the ribs to the pelvis in front, c) the deeper aspect of the rectus sheath leading to the diaphragm and the psoas muscles. This is part of the Deep Front Line. (See figure 7.4b to see these cords in cross section.)

The diaphragm is tied to the pelvis in many ways – muscularly through the quadratus lumborum, psoas complex, abdominal obliques and the rectus abdominis itself. But if we change our focus from these muscles and look instead to the fascia surrounding them, we see four cords which are essential to balance.

Just outside the rectus abdominis is a fascial strip called the *semi-lunar line* – marked as 'aponeurosis of internal oblique muscle' in figure 7.5 – where the three layers of the two obliques and the transversus abdominis seal together before splitting around the rectus abdominis itself. While balance of the muscles is important, getting an even tone in this semi-lunar line is also important. This fascial line runs from the outside of the pubic tubercle to the seventh rib cartilage. It can be felt as a 'valley' between the outside edges of the rectus abdominis and the muscle of the obliques.

The corresponding set of cords in the back are shorter and stronger, but just as important. The lateral raphe is a thick band of fascia that runs from the eleventh and twelfth ribs down to the iliac crest laterally to the quadratus lumborum. It could be said to be part of the thoracolumbar fascia, and it is associated with the widest muscle of the erector spinae, the iliocostalis lumborum, as well as the quadratus lumborum and the transversus abdominis. Again, this is where the various fascial layers seal into one, providing a strong and stable link between the ribs and pelvis in back.

These four cords, the two semi-lunar in front and the lateral raphes behind, are fascial sealing lines and mark the general division line between the Lateral Line to the outside of these cords and the Superficial Front Line, Deep Front Line and Superficial Back Line, which run medial to them but each line taking up a different layer of depth in the body, on either side of the sagittal plane.

In hyperlordotic or swayback patterns, or in those where the rib cage has dropped behind the pelvis, the posterior cords of the lateral raphe are likely to be shorter and require lengthening, while the front cords will often be eccentrically taut. In flexed or collapsed patterns, the anterior cords will be relatively shorter than the back (they are always absolutely longer, since the pelvis dips and the rib cage rises in the front – we are talking about relative balance, not the same metric).

In side-bending patterns, of course, the two left cords, front and back, could be shorter than their corresponding right cords.

In rotational patterns, such as rotoscoliosis, the contralateral cords will be tight; in other words, the left posterior and the right anterior, or vice-versa. It is, of course, possible to have a rotational pattern along with either a hyperlordotic or collapsed posture, expanding the number of possible patterns to eight, with subtle variations based on individual movement patterns.

Fat Distribution around the Lumbar Spine

'Why am I soft in the middle? The rest of my life is so hard!' – Paul Simon

Given that the middle of the body in some of us is carrying a bit of extra weight, the best way for the body's structure to carry that weight is as a 'spare tire' – distributed evenly between front and back. We all know large people who can dance us under the table; their weight seems only to lubricate their movement, not to inhibit it. If you observe those people, however overweight they may be according to the President's Council on Physical Fitness, you will see that their weight is balanced front and back around the spine.

Having short cords in back often accompanies a 'bay window' or beer belly – in other words, a pattern of fat that hangs off the front of the body. This pattern is much harder on the body's structure, pulling on the neck, compressing the low back, and requiring more tightness in the back of the legs. Lengthening the cords of the lateral raphes in the back will go a long way – over time – toward the more balanced 'spare tire', even if no weight is actually lost.

Inter-Organ 'Joints'

The abdomino-pelvic cavity between the respiratory and pelvic diaphragms is a literally slippery area, where there are a whole series of 'joints' we have not considered at all – the interfaces between the organs. Every time you breathe, the organs have to slide on each other like two plates of wet glass; adhesions caused by infection, trauma or disuse can inhibit these small but important 'joints'. This important relation between the fascial sacs for the organs and the body wall of the abdominal balloon is well treated in the books of Jean-Pierre Barrall (1996) and Peter Schwind (2006). These techniques are beyond the scope of this volume.

Nevertheless, getting the muscular belts of the abdominal balloon and the fascial cords of the parachute balanced will go a long way toward getting this complex area under the easy control of your clients, to the benefit of the pelvis and legs below, and the rib cage, shoulders and neck above. It is to the rib cage and respiration, which occupies the northern half of the ventral cavity, that we now turn our attention.

The Rib Basket

The entire ventral cavity is largely concerned with chemical exchange with the outside world. It is an unalterable fact of living creatures: if they are to continue to go uphill against entropy, then they must bring 'stuff' in from the outside world and make it their own, and export other stuff out as now useless waste. In the lower half of the ventral cavity, we looked at the muscles that surround the alimentary canal and kidneys. These organs are largely responsible for bringing in the fuel and the building blocks of life, and getting rid of the chemistry the body can no longer use.

Housed in the upper half of this large opening is a central pump that moves this freight to and from all the cells, and special bellows that filter out particular gases that require a faster exchange than the alimentary canal allows – in other words, the heart and lungs.

The heart requires protection and a steady base from which to work, and the lungs require a constantly variable change of pressure, up and down. The structures evolved to meet those contrasting needs are the ribs and sternum, bent and sprung into the truss of the thoracic spine. The heart sits in a tough set of bags slung between the more fixed points of the posterior breastbone and the anterior part of the spine. The sponges of the lungs sit on either side, slung vertically between the neck and lower back, being alternately stretched and compressed by the highly mobile ribs. The individual and collective mobility of the ribs suggests that the word 'rib cage' might be a useful thought for the heart, but we suggest the image of your mother's old wicker laundry basket is more appropriate for the way the ribs surround the lungs.

The Ribs in Four Sections

This rib basket can be usefully divided into four sections. Taking it from the bottom, the lowest three ribs form a useful section that relates the ribs to the hips. At least two, and sometimes all three, of these ribs are floating ribs, with free distal ends. This extra freedom permits more movement, which is of great benefit because the abdominal muscles, especially the two obliques, link these ribs to the pelvis, allowing or restraining the twisting and leaning motions that take place between these two large blocks.

These 'pelvic' ribs surround the kidneys, and are associated with them and the adrenal glands that sit atop the kidneys.

The next functional division of the rib basket consists of a set of four ribs – all connected to the subcostal cartilage – which we will term the *abdominal ribs*. While these ribs are not as free as the floating ribs, the large cartilage breastplate allows a lot of movement. These ribs exhibit a strong 'bucket handle' effect, expanding out to the side on the inhalation. These ribs surround the stomach and spleen on the left and the liver on the right, and are associated with the glands of the pancreas and liver, and the small xiphoid point of the sternal dagger.

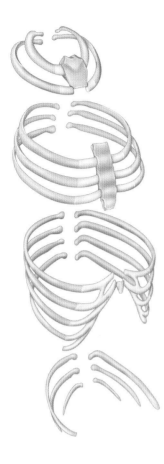

Figure 7.7: The rib 'basket' can be seen in four major functional sections: the first two neck ribs, the next three chest ribs, the next four abdominal ribs, and the final three pelvic ribs.

The next section is ribs three–five, all of which tie directly into the body of the sternum, thus making these ribs more stable. They surround the heart itself (and are thus associated with the thymus), and make a strong connection between the mediastinum and the shoulders. The pectoralis minor – the major tether for scapular movement – attaches to these ribs. While still mobile, these ribs have more stabilizing duties than the ribs below them.

The final section of the ribs is the upper two. These ribs are flatter, smaller and even more stable than the rest of the ribs below. Both of these attach into the handle of the sternal dagger, the manubrium. They are known here as the *neck ribs*, since, via the scalene muscles, they provide a stable base for neck movements and for controlling the heavy head atop the delicate neck. These ribs are associated with the thyroid gland.

Ribs and the Spine

If we take a look around the back to see how the ribs are attached to the spine, we find a very interesting pattern. At one point in our evolution we may have had three pairs of ribs, similar in formation to a six-rayed starfish, anterior, transverse and posterior. The posterior ribs bent together at the back to form the neural arch and the spinous processes. The transverse ribs became the transverse processes. The anterior ribs remain as our ribs, but, reflecting the old pattern, they are bent around the front of the transverse processes to put the rib heads up against the discs – at least, in ribs 2 to 9.

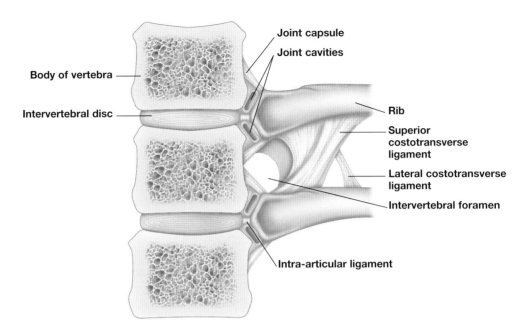

Body of vertebra

Intervertebral disc

Joint capsule

Joint cavities

Rib

Superior costotransverse ligament

Lateral costotransverse ligament

Intervertebral foramen

Intra-articular ligament

Figure 7.8: The rib heads attach to the transverse processes on their way to a complex and interesting joint with the corresponding disc, and the two vertebral bodies on either side of it.

This means that a complete movement of the ribs in breathing acts to hydrate the discs and keep them healthy. For so many of us, our perception of the ribs stops somewhere around to the side, and does not extend into the back, where the complete movement of the ribs really contributes to our long-term health. The work described here can help with enhancing movement in the front of the ribs, and Chapter 8 also contains techniques which will help engender this awareness and movement where the ribs meet the spine.

Accessory Muscles of Breathing

The principal muscle for breathing is of course the *diaphragm*, to which we will turn our attention in a moment. Several other muscles surround the rib basket and help (or hinder) breathing. Let us look at those first.

The abdominal obliques hold the pelvic and abdominal ribs to the pelvis, and thus they provide a steady base for the initial part of diaphragmatic movement, though they must relent in the latter stage to allow the ribs to rise. In this author's opinion, standing tension in the rectus abdominis runs counter to easy and complete breathing, but there are as many theories of the 'proper breath' as there are people to espouse them.

The quadratus lumborum provides a direct extension of the diaphragm from the twelfth rib to the pelvis, and can inhibit deep breathing in the back if is too tight or (more often) too fascially short.

The serratus posterior superior and the serratus posterior inferior are often listed as breathing assistants. The muscular elements of these fascial retinacula are so diminutive as to leave us wondering whether they really have much effect on breathing. The levatores costarum (which we will examine more closely in Chapter 8) are likewise listed as breathing assistants. Again, it is doubtful that they exert much motive power on the ribs – though when they spasm, they certainly do cause a catch in the breath.

Of course, other accessory muscles can be used in breathing if it is for some reason difficult: the sternocleidomastoid, the pectoral muscles, and the erector muscles of the back can all help in extremis. The principal muscles assisting the diaphragm, though, are the scalenes and the intercostals.

The intercostals are commonly thought to draw the ribs together in the inhale, but putting your fingertips between the ribs and doing a strong inhale will soon put paid to that notion. The ribs

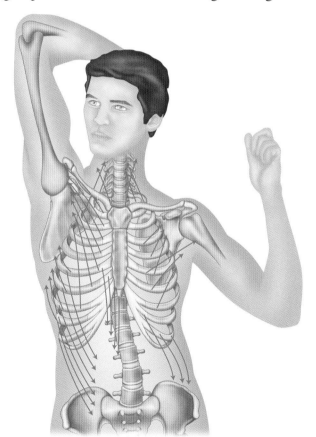

really do not get closer to each other, even in a strong inhale; nor do they spread during the exhale. If the intercostals are active in breathing, it is to slide the ribs obliquely along each other. This author follows Jon Zahourek (private correspondence) in seeing the intercostals primarily as muscles of walking – winding and unwinding the torso's rotation with each step.

Figure 7.9: The many muscles around the rib cage can assist with breathing when required, or inhibit breathing if they are too tight and short.

That leaves us with the scalenes. These are widely seen these days as the secondary muscles of breathing, leaving the intercostals as tertiary. The scalenes surround the transverse processes of the second through the sixth cervical vertebrae, coming down to the first and second ribs like a skirt around the neck. In breathing, they lift the upper two ribs, or prevent them from being pulled down.

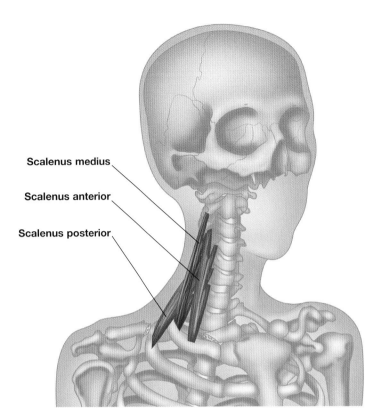

Scalenus medius

Scalenus anterior

Scalenus posterior

Figure 7.10: The scalenes form a skirt around the neck from the first and second ribs. The middle and posterior scalenes moderate side-to-side movement of the head, as well as assisting in breathing. The anterior scalene can really pull the cervical vertebrae down and forward in dysfunction.

In dysfunction, we should divide the middle and posterior scalenes (which are incompletely separate muscles in any case) from the anterior. The middle and posterior muscles are paravertebral, and therefore act as 'the quadratus lumborum of the neck', creating – or more often preventing/stabilizing – lateral flexion of the neck.

The anterior scalene runs more anteriorly from the anterior tubercles of the third through the sixth cervical vertebrae down and forward to the first rib – thus qualifying it more as 'the psoas of the neck'. It is designed to use the neck as an origin and the ribs as an insertion, pulling up on the ribs during inhalation. If you push your sternocleidomastoid out of the way medially and place your finger pads on the slick, dense muscle beneath it and breathe in, you will feel the anterior scalene tighten, either all the way through the breath, or right at the top of the breath at least.

Unfortunately, the neck is not the most stable of organs, especially if the suboccipital muscles start to shorten (as they often do in sustained fear patterns – see Chapter 8). Too often, the anterior scalene shortens to pull the neck down to the ribs; it should be opened in cases of head-forward posture, or its variant, a posteriorly tilted rib cage.

The Diaphragm

This leaves us with the diaphragm, the undisputed primary muscle of breathing. One only has to get the 'wind knocked out' by a blow to the xiphoid area to realize how useless the other muscles of breathing are without the diaphragm.

The diaphragm is a large umbrella whose stem is comprised of two crura that attach to the front of the lumbar spine, and whose edge is attached to the xiphoid and all the way around the lower margins of the ribs. Its movement is remarkably similar to that of a jellyfish.

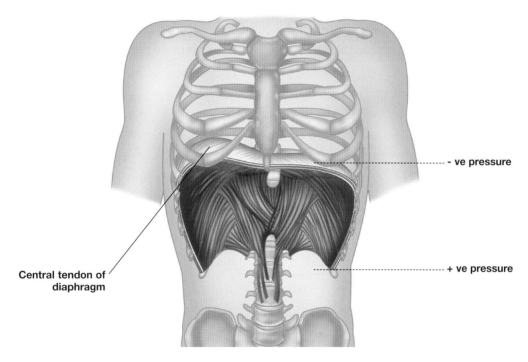

Figure 7.11: The diaphragm is a double dome – one under each lung – that moves down on the inhalation and recoils back up on the outbreath. The pressure is always positive below it and negative above it.

The diaphragm is a thin but remarkably strong muscle that lies poised between the digestive organs of the abdominal cavity and the heart and lungs of the thoracic cavity. The word 'poised' is appropriate at the bottom of the breath, in that the positive pressure from the lower cavity (which is there no matter how you starve or purge yourself) is balanced by the suction and negative pressure from the spongy lungs (which always want to collapse, no matter how far you breathe out).

In a four-legged creature, the diaphragm pumps backward and forward, obliquely to gravity. In us, it pumps up and down more or less in the gravity line. The pressure in the pelvic cavity is strongly positive. It is less so in the abdominal cavity, and in the thoracic cavity it is negative, leaving the diaphragm cleverly poised in the middle at the zero point.

Although we used the image of an umbrella above, the diaphragm is best seen as a double dome, one under each lung, with a central tendon running from the center of one dome to the other under the heart. This central portion of the diaphragm develops with the heart essentially 'above the head' in the embryo's septum transversum, and is folded down into the chest in a unique piece of developmental origami. So it cannot move down very far without pulling on the pericardial bag around the heart. Therefore this center point of the diaphragm only moves down about one and one-quarter centimeters (half an inch) for most people, though it can be trained by singers, divers and yoga practitioners to move four times that distance.

The two domes under the lungs, however, move down several inches (again, dependent on activity and training), pulling air into the lungs above each dome, and acting like a piston in the middle of the ventral cavity to move all the organs. While the heart, safe in its triangular housing and attached to the sternum and thoracic spine, escapes being moved much, the liver and stomach both move down and together, the kidneys ride up and down the psoas, and the intestines roll and unroll in the wake of the diaphragmatic pulse. Even the lungs themselves rotate a little within the ribs as the forces change and pull them open.

Diaphragmatic Movement

It is essential to understand that the diaphragmatic fibers are mostly vertical. Most of the muscle fibers of the body are either directly along the line of the body or slightly oblique to it. The diaphragm is widely thought of as a horizontal muscle, but in fact the horizontal part is the central tendon, the connective tissue under the lungs and heart. The majority of the muscle fibers are on the sides of the domes, and therefore for the most part act vertically.

This puts the diaphragm in the unique position of being a muscle that regularly switches the origin for the insertion in the middle of its movement. At the beginning of the inhale, when the diaphragmatic fibers contract, the lower rim of the ribs and the lumbar spine is the origin, and the central tendon is the insertion. The central tendon is pulled down, stretching the lungs down also and pulling air into them. As the tops of the domes move down, the organs of the abdominal balloon move down with them, compressing the abdomen. Fluid-filled organs can only compress a little bit, and soon the central tendon is pulled down against the resistant, fluid-filled balloon. Since it cannot be pushed any farther down, at this point in the breath the origin and insertion reverse. The central tendon, resting on the abdomen, becomes the origin, and the vertical fibers, continuing to contract, act to pull the lower rim of the rib basket up. In most breathing patterns, the scalenes assist from above to lift the upper ribs.

You can feel this shift in yourself or in others by putting your hands on ribs 6 to 9 (the easy place your hands will go on the sides) and listening to a few breath cycles. Breathing patterns differ, but in most people there will be two distinct phases of the inhale. The early part will have the ribs more still, and in the second half they will move up (and out, figure 7.12) more strongly.

The transition may be more gradual or even indiscernible in those with a trained breath for singing or yoga, but nevertheless you will realize that they are moving differently at the end of the breath than at the beginning.

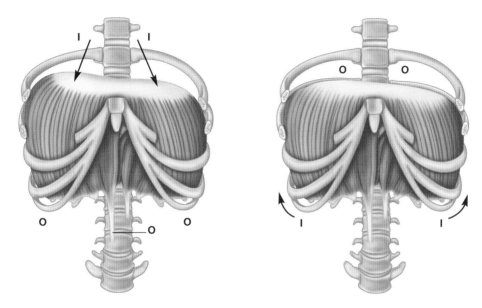

Figure 7.12a & b: The diaphragm switches its origin and insertion in the middle of its contraction; a) At first the ribs form the origin, and the centers of the domes are pulled down, b) in the second half of the inhalation, the central tendon becomes the origin, and the contraction of the diaphragm lifts the ribs.

This second movement of the diaphragm, pulling up on the ribs, is primarily and paradoxically responsible for the expansion of the rib basket, both from side to side and front to back – both the 'bucket handle' movement of the ribs out to the side and the 'pump handle' movement of the ribs moving away from the thoracic spine in front. The diaphragm itself is pulling up and in on the ribs; yet the box expands in these two ways because of the way the ribs are shaped and sprung, not because the ribs are being pulled out and up by muscles outside the ribs, even though they may help. The primary movement that powers the inhalation is the diaphragm.

The exhalation is said to be a natural process of elastic recoil in the lungs, requiring no action at all, but very few people have a contraction-free inhale in our speeded-up Western society. Who can wait that long, for the natural exhalationto happen? Assess your clients for excess contraction on the exhale, and do what you can to make it lighter and less effortful.

The other exhalation problem frequently encountered but hard to see is that the diaphragm fails to fully relax at the bottom of the exhale. Many people, especially if they are anxious, tend to retain some tension in the diaphragm all the time, so it never fully relaxes, never fully expels the air. Tracking the outbreath and using your hands to assist a full relaxation of the diaphragm is a service to all the regulatory systems of your client's body – neural and organic, as well as musculoskeletal.

Breath flows in and out of the body approximately twenty-thousand times per day. To call it the river of life is no exaggeration, though it more resembles the tide, ebbing and flowing. In any case, it is the essential and central movement on which so many others are built. Small aberrations in the breathing pattern – repeated so many times per day, so many days in a row, right in the middle of the Deep Front Line and the organic self – can lead to many imbalances. The converse is also true: getting the breathing to take a more balanced path can make diverse problems disappear as the body rights itself.

BodyReading the Abdomen, Thorax, and Breathing

So, it seems there are as many opinions about the breath as there are teachers talking about it. What constitutes the perfect breath is more likely determined not by some dictated fixed idea, but rather the ability to match the needs and demands of any given activity, whether that be marathon running, yoga practice or television watching. Our idea of the perfect breath is that it is simply present and responsive throughout the trunk: front, back and sides.

The ribs are clearly designed to move, pump-handle fashion in the upper four, basket-handle fashion in seven to ten, with five and six having a little of both up and outward movements. The shoulders should also move up and out in a relaxed fashion with a full inhalation in scale with the upward and outward excursion of the ribs.

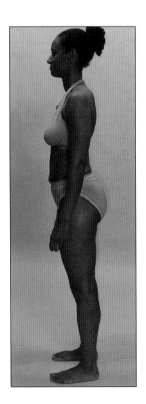

Full analysis of the breath cycle takes time and the ability to compare real people, which is limited in this context, but we encourage you to look for certain elements. Our aim for the trunk is to have the diaphragm, the principal muscle of breathing, aligned over the lower diaphragm of the pelvic floor; the more engaged they are, the healthier the reciprocal interaction between them. In Chapter 6 we balanced the pelvis above the feet, and now we aim to put the diaphragm on top of that. This will require balance front and back, in the four pillars or cords mentioned above, side to side between the two lateral lines and the sternum, in line with the symphysis pubis by balancing the abdominal 'X' of the obliques.

Figure 7.13: In this lady's structure you can see that her pelvic floor is aiming up and forward and her diaphragm is aiming down and forward. The meeting point of what should be two opposing forces is just in front of her abdomen. We need to bring more reciprocation to this relationship, by balancing the four pillars described, as well as lengthening and releasing her hip flexors.

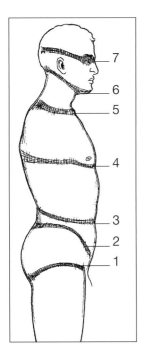

Another common issue that can restrict the breath is the horizontal band that often develops around the level of the fifth rib. This is one of a series of bands that were described by Schultz and Feitis (1996) and pictured in the diagram left.

This line is a natural indentation, because it marks the transition between the attachments of the rectus abdominis and the pectoralis major, but the tissue should still move over the ribs, both in breathing and active movement. Make a basic assessment of this area by asking your client to bring their arms over their head and extend them backwards (as far as is comfortable and safe to do so) or to side-bend to both sides. In these tests it is not range of motion that we are interested in as much as the quality of the movement of the tissue over the skeleton.

Figure 7.14: The horizontal bands described by Schultz and Feitis.

Another common pattern includes tilts of the rib cage to one side. For this you need to lift and lengthen the shorter side, spreading the tissue of the longer abdominal obliques and going into the deeper layers of tissue to get to the short quadratus lumborum if necessary. Psoas major can also be involved in tilts of the thorax, pulling the twelfth rib and diaphragm toward the shorter side.

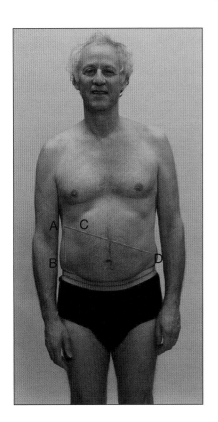

The psoas major is also often implicated in rotations of the rib cage, pulling it to turn away from the shortened side. Before dealing with this deep tissue, though, we need to address the more superficial level of the obliques, lengthening the diagonal from one anterior superior iliac spine to the ribs on the opposite side of the trunk.

Figure 7.15: This gentleman demonstrates (A–B) right tilt of the rib cage, so we would work to lift his right lateral tissue (eventually followed by his right psoas and quadratus lumborum) and spread his left. He also appears to show a rotation to the left, as the line from his right costal arch to his left ASIS (C–D) appears shorter than the same line on the opposite side.

Abdomen and Thorax Techniques

Rectus Abdominis and Sternocostal Fascia (SFL)

As part of the Superficial Front Line, the fascia of the rectus abdominis is continuous with the sternocleidomastoid. It can therefore be involved in drawing the head forward into an anterior shift if it is pulled down because of an anterior tilt in the pelvis or overly tight abdomen or even, as in this model, hip flexors.

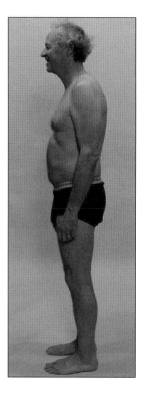

Figure 7.16: In the side view of the same model, we can see how the tissue over the sternum is being drawn inferiorly, even as far as the front of the pelvis. Following this line up the body, we can see how it relates to the anterior shift of the head.

Begin the stroke above the pubic hair, or higher if it is more appropriate for your client. Have your fingers curled to sink into the layer of the rectus abdominis, and then uncurl them using your finger extensors to engage the tissue and stretch it away from the pelvis. Dropping your elbows allows you to remain at the level of the muscle without diving deeper into the abdomen itself, which could cause pain and impingement of the more fragile underlying tissue.

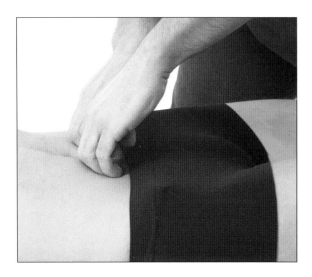

Figure 7.17: Using the uncurling of your fingers and dropping your elbows creates a scooping action to engage the tissue at the correct level.

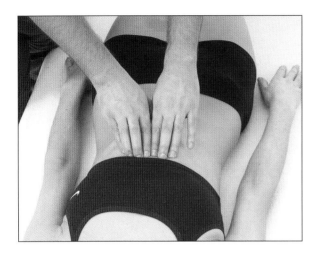

Figure 7.18: Continue the stroke along the length of the rectus abdominis, releasing and re-engaging when the adipose tissue restricts your ability to maintain the connection.

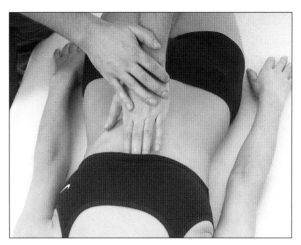

Figure 7.19: Dropping your elbows again to scoop the tissue over the ribs avoids pressing into the bone or cartilage. Avoid the xiphoid process, but carry the stroke further along the sternum.

Many people will benefit from all of this tissue being lifted. It can be informative for their structure to carry this stroke through from close to the pubic attachment all the way to the top of the sternum. Rarely will you be able to manage it in one continuous stroke, as the adipose tissue tends to build up, and for ladies the bra strap will create a barrier – so bringing your hands off and then re-engaging a little lower than where you left off will effectively draw the tissue superiorly.

Working underneath the bra strap may be outside the boundaries of your professional code. If so, then avoid it. But once the intention is clarified with the client and she realizes the breast tissue will not be invaded upon, then she will likely be comfortable with this technique.

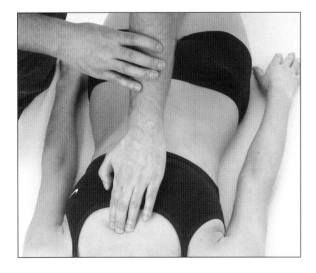

Figure 7.20: Work along the sternum itself and the tissue either side to release around the sternocostal joints.

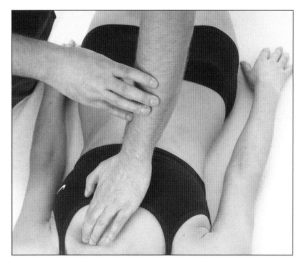

Figure 7.21: As we reach the top of the sternum, carrying the intention out toward the arm can help open the chest. Do not follow through onto the throat.

Side-Lying Thorax (LTL)

To lift the lateral tissue of a shortened side, sink into the tissue just above the level of the iliac crest and, by dropping your elbows, carry the deep investing layer superiorly. Carry your connection over the rib cage and, taking care neither to press too hard into the lateral ribs nor simply to skim over the top with the skin and adipose tissue; use the sense in your hands to engage the layers of myofascia in between and carry them up.

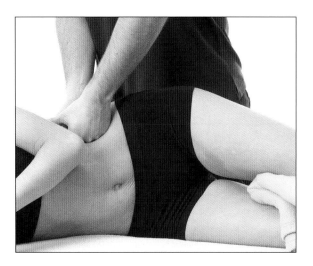 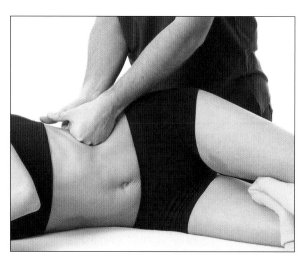

Figure 7.22a & b: A scooping action of the forearms can carry the fascial tissue superiorly, lengthening the Lateral Line.

The tissue on the opposite, longer lateral aspect could be 'locked long' and therefore in need of transverse rather than longitudinal work. Such spreading of the tissue can also be very useful for clients with limited lateral movement of the ribs during inhalation.

When working across the thorax we need to raise our shoulder girdle over the top of the client and use the back of our soft fists with our arms crossed. Alternatively we can use the heels of the hands as they engage the client's tissue and drop our bodyweight toward the massage couch to perform the stroke. The client is encouraged to breathe throughout the intervention to maintain a positive pressure in the thorax to work against, giving them better feedback and you more effective results.

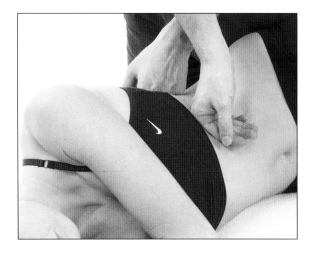

Figure 7.23: Spreading the tissue of the locked long side can help release any restrictions that may have developed because of fascial holding. Asking your client to 'breathe into my contact' can help open the tissue further, letting them do the work from the inside rather than forcing the tissue from outside.

External and Internal Obliques 'X' (SPL)

With the client supine but with their knees bent, start your engagement medially and slightly superiorly to the ASIS. Use the same method of contacting the tissue as above for the rectus fascia – extending your fingers into the fascial sheet – but this time angle your stroke toward the opposite ribs, following the line of the internal to external oblique muscles and eventually their connection into the serratus anterior.

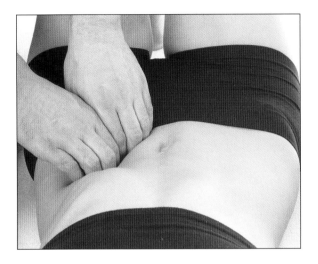 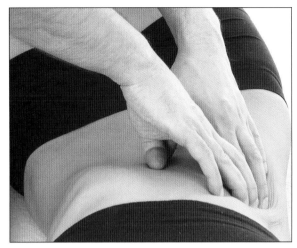

Figure 7.24a & b: For the obliques begin your contact just medially to the ASIS. Your stroke is heading toward the opposite costal margin and the serratus anterior.

The technique can be performed passively, with just the breath acting as movement, or the client can drop their knees toward the side on which you are standing; this will help draw the ASIS away from the opposite ribs. Another possibility would be to have the client reach across their body with the arm on the same side as you are standing, to create a stretch by taking the ribs on the opposite side away from the ASIS.

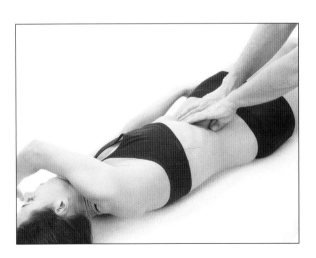

Figure 7.25: To assist the stretch, the client can drop their knees to the same side you are working from or reach their arm away from you. Extend the stroke over the ribs to the interface between the external obliques and the serratus anterior (if comfortable to do so, it could be extended further onto the tissue of the serratus anterior).

Ensure the completeness of the stroke by following it all the way through to the point at which the serratus anterior and external obliques meet and, depending on the client's pattern, carry the stroke into the tissue of this shoulder stabilizing muscle.

Side-Lying Internal and External Obliques (LTL)

The tissue on the side of the body is often imbalanced due to issues between the front and back of the body. We can work the lines of the obliques in order to create more length in any that appear short. Using the curled finger technique as shown previously (as with the rectus abdominis and oblique 'X'), you can work from the PSIS toward the front of the ribs for the internal oblique fibers while the client reaches forward with their upper arm. This technique corrects the more common pattern of the rib cage falling behind the pelvis.

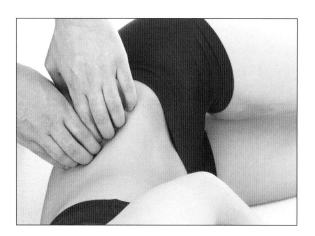
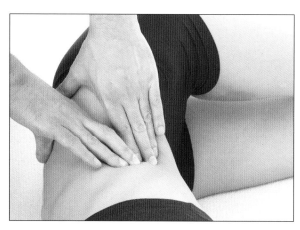

Figure 7.26a & b: Have the client's hips flexed to help stabilize the pelvis as the client reaches forward with the upper arm.

To contact the external obliques, use the same technique but come from above the ASIS toward the back of the rib cage as the client reaches back with their upper arm. This addresses the less common pattern where the rib cage is held in front of the pelvis.

You can add further accuracy by engaging your contact at the correct layer, in the same way as for the 'cleaning the edges of the ilium (LTL)' technique shown in Chapter 6, page 137.

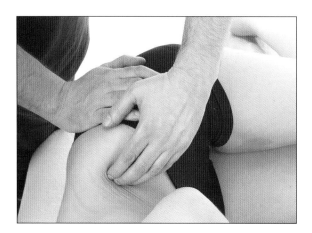
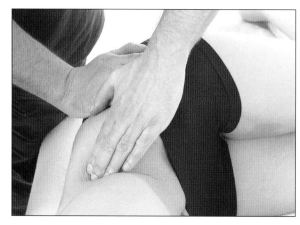

Figure 7.27a & b: Use your body behind the client or your non-working hand to stabilize the pelvis as the client reaches back.

Lateral Raphe Lift (SBL and LTL)

With your client flexed forward on the bench, kneel behind them and sink your fingertips into the tissue lateral to the erector muscles. Ask your client to then slowly roll back up into sitting whilst you lift the tissue, gliding toward the twelfth rib. This is an ideal movement for helping correct posteriorly tilted rib cages, when this line of fascia will be shortened. Several repetitions of this technique are often required, within a session or over several sessions, to release the heavy fascia of the lateral raphe.

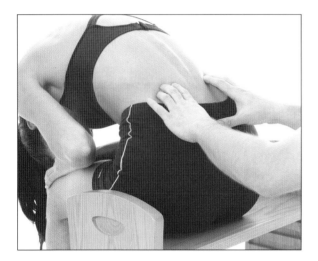 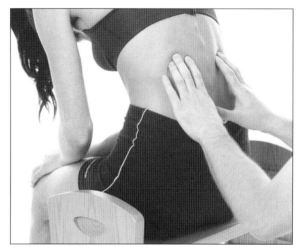

Figure 7.28a & b: Kneeling behind the seated client have them roll forward and then engage the tissue lateral to the erector spinae with your fingers and, keeping them and your wrists straight, slowly lift the tissue as the client slowly unfurls to sit upright. Position your hands and fingers such they unroll around them into easy upright sitting, neither flexed nor hyperextended in the lumbar spine.

Intercostal and Fifth Rib Line (LTL)

The Schultz band (figure 7.14) that often develops along the line of the fifth rib can be opened along the side using a soft spreading technique (figure 7.29). Have the client breathe up into the area between the opposing hands to aid the release of the tissue.

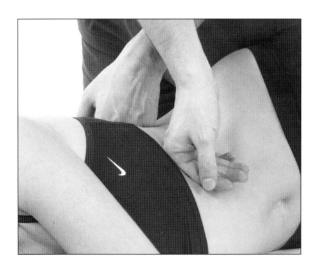

Figure 7.29: The back of the hands can be used to mold to the rib cage, engaging the first layer of tissue that feels locked or tight. As the client breathes up into the lateral ribs, the tissue can be spread by dropping your bodyweight over the top of your hands.

To work with more precision through the fifth rib band and to release between the ribs to access any of the intercostals that appear to be restricted, use your fingertips between the ribs. You can sink into the deeper layers of tissue this time, as you have the advantage of a sharper tool to use, but still clear the area one layer at a time, working from superficial to deep.

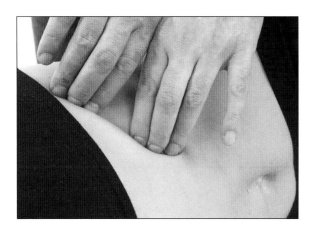

Figure 7.30: Swim your fingers between the ribs and ask your client to breathe up to your fingers (which can serve as a simple awareness exercise for your client as well). As the lung pressure increases you can then glide through the intercostal tissue, spreading your fingertips by rolling the MCP joints of your index fingers together for greater precision with less effort.

This technique can be useful not only for restricted breath but also in cases of limited rotation when walking, as it allows the ribs to move again, giving back to the rib cage the ability to wind and unwind during the gait cycle (see 'Accessory Muscles of Breathing', page 166).

Costal Arch Cleaning (SFL and LTL)

Adhesions and restrictions often form in the area along the costal arch. Deeper fascial layers of the abdominal muscles attach onto it, the superficial layers pass over it, the fascial extensions of the diaphragm attach deep to it – thus, there are many different directions of force at various degrees of depth. The tissue will also be drawn in different directions depending on any tilt or shift of the rib cage.

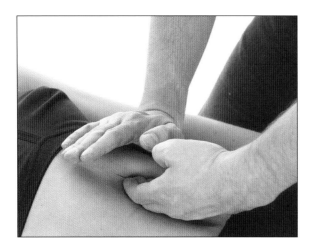 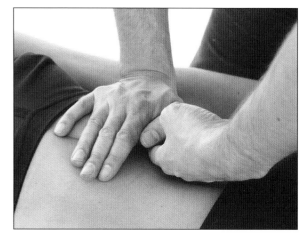

Figure 7.31a & b: The upper hand is lifted slightly in (a) to illustrate the hand positioning. It then supports the ribs, (b) pressing the tissue into the working fingers of the lower hand, which can then take the tissue in an anterior or posterior direction.

With the rectus abdominis and abdominal 'X' techniques, you should already have cleared much of the superficial tissue, allowing you to now work along the attachments of the arch. The most common direction to take them is posteriorly, due to the higher incidence of posterior tilt of the thorax, which will project the lower ribs forward.

Use your 'head' hand to support the ribs from above, pressing into them slightly to give some ease to the tissue, which the fingers of the 'foot' hand can then engage, drawing the tissue back following the line of the arch.

Diaphragm Release (DFL)

Using the same hand positions (figure 7.31a & b), this time using a little more slack in the rib cage, can allow the fingers of the working hand to sink under the anterior ribs just lateral to the rectus abdominis and curl onto the posterior aspect of the arch. How far you can reach is dependent on the openness of the tissue, but you will probably not be on the muscle fibers themselves, but almost certainly on the fascial attachments of the diaphragm.

Make sure that you curl your fingers under the arch by rolling off it and not by diving deep at an angle from the abdomen, as this could lead you to impinging visceral tissue instead. Ask your client to let you know if they feel sharp, burning or stabbing pain, which can be an indication that you are pinching visceral tissue.

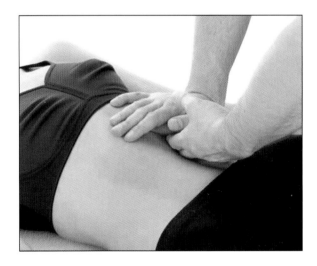

Figure 7.32: Notice the low angle of the forearm, which allows the fingers of the working hand to be almost parallel with the rib cage and thereby not press into the abdomen.

Once your hands are in position, you can simply draw the tissue in whichever direction is required by moving your arm to guide your wrist forward or back. The fascia of the diaphragm may also need to be drawn superiorly, by extending your fingers up along the anterior surface of the rib cage, or inferiorly, by flexing your fingertips into the tissue and slowly withdrawing your hand from below the thorax.

The goal of these techniques is not a 'perfect' breath, but a free and easy ebb and flow that supports all of our other activities. Remember, as a practitioner, to keep your own breath free and easy as you work. You are unlikely to get relaxed breathing in the client if you are puffing or straining or locking your breath in the process of doing these techniques. Getting totally relaxed in the performance of these strokes is time well invested, not only in terms of your own career longevity and health, but also in the results obtained for your client.

Encouraging the Exhale

Often we find it necessary to balance the exhalation with the inhalation for those people who appear to breathe in further than they exhale, rarely letting the rib cage fully deflate. Have the client lie on their side and, standing at their back, place your cephalad hand around the scapula, acromion process, and clavicle of the uppermost shoulder girdle. Your other hand spans the lateral aspect of the rib cage just below the level of the breast tissue if working with a female client. This position allows you to depress the upper ribs via the shoulder girdle by pressing down on with the upper hand and the middle and lower ribs using the thenar and then hypothenar aspects of your lower hand in turn.

Encourage the client to inhale, and as they exhale slowly depress the sections of the ribs in turn, starting with the upper ribs, then moving to the middle ribs, and finishing with the lower ribs. Pause when the exhalation is complete, and then give gentle resistance against the expansion of the ribs for the subsequent inhalation. Follow the reverse order, lower, middle and then upper ribs, gradually releasing most of the pressure but not all, to maintain some degree of inward force on the lungs when they are reinflated.

As the client exhales again try to deepen the exhalation by taking up more of the slack in the movement of the ribs, before releasing to allow for the inhalation. This cycle can be followed four or five times, with each exhalation becoming increasingly fuller.

Please note: Do not perform this technique if there is any doubt over the health of the ribs and costal area, and/or presence of osteoporosis or osteopenia.

The Spine

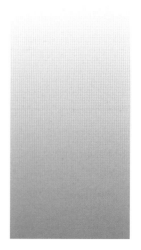

8

Behind the ventral cavity lies the complex anatomy of the spine that surrounds the dorsal cavity. Since we are focusing on the fascial and myofascial anatomy, we will use this opportunity to point out only a few salient features of the osseous and ligamentous layout of the spine, moving onto the muscles that stabilize and move it.

The vertebral column is divided into two sections, fore and aft: the bodies and discs anterior to the spinal cord, and the neural arch that runs around and behind it.

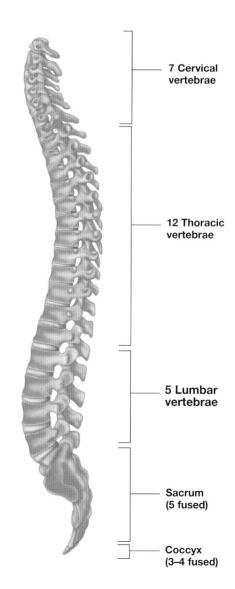

7 Cervical vertebrae

12 Thoracic vertebrae

5 Lumbar vertebrae

Sacrum (5 fused)

Coccyx (3–4 fused)

Figure 8.1: The spinal cord divides the spine into an anterior column (the bodies and discs of the original notochord) and a posterior truss work (the neural arch, bristling with its many processes).

The Anterior Column: The Primacy of the Discs

Taking the anterior column of the discs and bodies first, most anatomies will start with the idea that the spine is a series of vertebrae with discs in between. The very opposite is the case: the spine is a series of discs with the vertebrae in between. This seemingly nonsensical distinction is worthwhile: whether considered phylogenetically or ontogenetically, the discs come first. The original spine was one long disc: a tough outer tunic that consisted of a series of fabric layers with fibers running in various directions – fibers spiraling left, spiraling right; longitudinal and circumferential fibers. Sealed within all these layers was a pulpy fluid center, making a strong whiplike armature for movement in the middle of the early chordates.

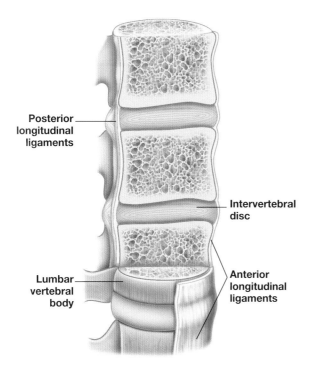

Posterior longitudinal ligaments

Intervertebral disc

Lumbar vertebral body

Anterior longitudinal ligaments

The bodies of the vertebrae specialize and develop out of this long disc (known as the *notochord*). The fascial collagen net of the disc's annular tunic is continuous with the collagen within the bone of the vertebral body, and thus no disc can 'slip'. Discs can break down, such that the pulpy center pushes out through the annular walls to create pressure on the nerves, but the disc cannot actually move relative to the vertebrae, because vertebral body and disc were made from the same original fibrous stuff.

Figure 8.2: The intervertebral disc is a piece of ancient construction that is subject to wear and tear in daily life as well as the shocks of injury.

The discs and bodies are covered up the front of the spine by the long, cohesive and very strong anterior longitudinal ligament (ALL). The ALL runs the entire length from the tailbone up to the bottom of the occiput, joining the entire spine and preventing excessive, spine-damaging extension. The ALL can shorten if held in a shortened position for a long time (as in a kyphosis), and it can be trained into becoming longer by strong spinal opening such as yoga backbend training.

A similarly strong but narrower ligament goes up behind the vertebral bodies and discs, the posterior longitudinal ligament (PLL). The PLL lies between the discs and the spinal cord, and prevents untoward flexion. It also prevents the discs from expanding backward into the spinal cord, although severe trauma can sometimes break this ligament and allow disc material to cause really severe damage to the spinal cord.

The area around the disc restrained by neither the ALL nor the PLL is the area most likely to see disc intrusion (figure 8.2). Unfortunately these two quadrants, left and right, are the areas where the spinal nerves exit from the spinal cord to the rest of the body. These nerve roots and horns are therefore the most likely to be pressured when the discs extrude.

This anterior part of the spine, if it could be considered separately, would essentially be a series of round spools with the tough but squishy discs in between. It could therefore be moved in any direction – flexed, extended, laterally flexed, rotated, circumducted – even including a small amount of axial extension and flexion (moving like an earthworm).

The Posterior Truss: The Slings and Arrows

Not so versatile in allowing movement is the posterior part of the spine – the neural arch and the many processes sticking out from the arch itself that provide attachments for the muscles and ligaments. The shapes of the interlocking facets between the vertebrae allow or disallow certain movements, as we will see just ahead.

The neural arch was built from two sets of 'ribs' – the transverse and posterior ribs – that were in the ancient proto-fish. The posterior ribs bent around toward each other until they formed an arch, and bound together in the back to form the spinous process. This process is still bifurcated in some vertebrae in some people, most commonly at C2, the axis.

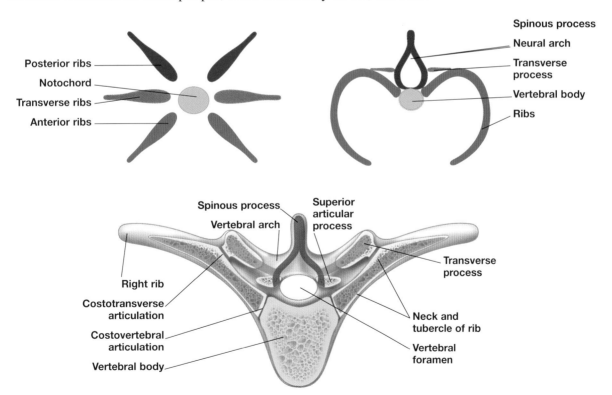

Figure 8.3: Two of the original three sets of ribs have converged to form the neural arch, the spinous processes and the transverse processes that form the principal places of muscle attachment in the spine.

The lateral transverse ribs formed the transverse processes. In our spine, these transverse processes separate the part of the neural arch between the body and transverse process (the *pedicle*) from the part between the transverse and spinous processes (the *lamina*).

The other processes sticking out from the vertebrae are the overlapping shingles of the articular processes. The two superior articular facets stick up, overlapping with the inferior articular facets of the vertebra above. This arrangement limits the mobility of the spine, but contributes greatly to its stability and smooth movement.

Tensegrity

This arrangement also contributes greatly to the spine's resilience. It is our contention that the bones of the spine essentially 'float' over each other. This is clear in the anterior part: each body floats on the disc below it. In the posterior part, the fact that these facet joints overlap like shingles gives the ligamentous capsules for these joints the opportunity to act as slings, where each successive vertebra is capable of 'floating' in the slings hanging from the upper edge of the facet joint of the vertebra below.

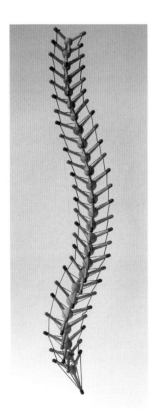
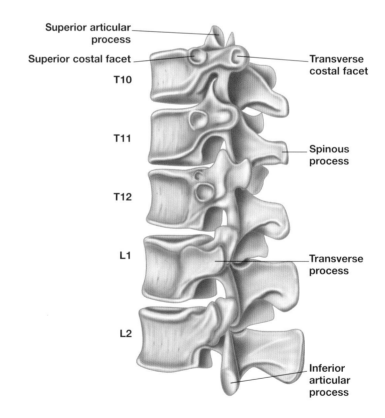

Figure 8.4: In (a), we see a tensegrity mast arranged somewhat like a spine. An essential element to this kind of mast is having a strut from the compression member (bone) above stick down below a strut coming up from the compression member below, with a tension member (wire, elastic or connective tissue) joining the two. You can see that arrangement in the model, and we see it in the anatomy also (b), where the superior articular facet reaches below the inferior articular facet of the vertebra above, and the two rest in the sling of the ligamentous capsule of the joint (model and photograph courtesy of Tom Flemons, www.intensiondesigns.com).

The name given to this kind of mechanics, where isolated compressional struts float balanced in a sea of tension, is *tensegrity* (as discussed in Chapter 1) – denoting that the integrity of such structures is determined by the relative balance among the tension members. To the degree that the spinal bones do float in this springy way, then all the muscles arrayed along the back of the spine have several possible jobs:

1) pull the spine into extension and create the secondary curves (more on this when we reach the muscles on page 189);
2) adjust the tensegrity in terms of direction, rotation and 'pre-stress' (this last term means to tighten the whole tensegrity of the spine so that it is more bouncy and can take more load without collapsing, or relax it for maximum mobility); or
3) pull the spinous processes together (which pulls the facets into the sling and then transfers the lift to the front of the vertebra like a pump handle, lifting the vertebra off the disc below it, minimizing the pressure down through the discs).

In dysfunction, excess tension in the muscles (including the muscles on the front of the spine like the psoas major) will pull the vertebrae together, collapsing this floating tensegrity into a stack of bricks. Ultimately, the discs do not appreciate being asked to act as bricks, and they break down. Asymmetrical tension will create both side-bends and rotations, pressuring discs and facets in particular places. Too little tension and the spine collapses forward, which simply exports the tension elsewhere, to the ribs, limbs and pelvis.

The Direction of the Facets
As well as being 'tension dependent', the facet joints line up in particular planes that allow or disallow movement. In the lumbar vertebrae (for brevity, we will take each section as a whole), the facets overlap in the sagittal plane. This arrangement allows easy flexion, extension and lateral flexion, but it severely limits rotation; when the lumbar vertebrae try to rotate, the facets run into each other. Although the sacro-lumbar joints allow a little more rotation, the rest of the lumbar vertebrae taken together account for only five degrees of rotation. This can be augmented slightly by flexing the lumbar spine before rotating, as the flexion pulls the facets apart from each other; hyperextension (lumbar lordosis) limits rotation even further, by pushing the lumbar facets together.

This arrangement makes for a strong hinging motion in the lower back (think how a dolphin moves) to transfer the force from the legs to the torso without dissipating that force in rotational movement.

Quite suddenly, at T12, the direction of the facets changes from the sagittal plane to a plane much closer to the frontal or coronal. The sternum in front and the spinous processes behind seriously limit the flexion and extension available in the thoracic area of the spine, but this shape of the facets allows significant rotational movement within the rib basket.

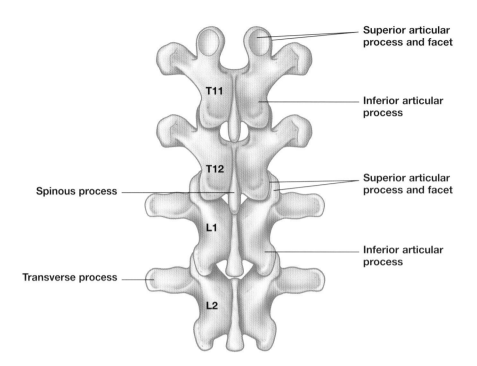

Figure 8.5: Below T12, the lumbar facets are located squarely in the sagittal plane, allowing all the motions but rotation. Above T12, they are located close to the frontal plane, allowing rotation and side-bending, but limited in flexion and extension.

This coronal orientation slowly tilts toward the horizontal as we move up the thoracic spine, such that by the time we reach the cervical section, the plane of the facets is approaching the transverse or horizontal. This process is complete by the time we reach the atlanto-axial and atlanto-occipital joints at the top, which are both quite close to the horizontal plane. These cervical facets thus allow every kind of motion – flexion, extension, side-bending and rotation – so that our head with its teleceptors is maximally mobile.

Thus we see a progression of the facet joint angles from oblique at the very bottom to sagittal to frontal to oblique to horizontal as we move up the spine. While the front of the spine is potentially totally mobile, the posterior part of the spine limits, and thus directs, movement.

Turning now to the larger processes that provide anchors for the spinal muscles, we see the series of spinous processes running along the back, and the series of transverse processes running along the left and right. These are joined by ligaments between and along the processes themselves: the intertransverse, interspinous and supraspinous ligaments.

The Pattern of the Musculature

Three basic single-segment muscles traverse these processes:

1) the intertransversarii, which express the pattern of transverse process to transverse process; these muscles create side-bending in concentric tension and prevent it in eccentric tension;
2) the interspinous muscles, which run from spinous process to spinous process, thus bringing the spinous processes together in spinal extension, or relaxing to let the spine fall into flexion; and
3) the rotators, which reach down and out from one spinous process to the transverse process of the vertebra below; these muscles create and modulate rotation.

These are the deepest and shortest muscles of the spine. They are not very powerful in muscular terms, but they neurologically *set* the tone and pattern of firing of the larger, more powerful muscles superficial to them. The latter basically follow the same patterning as these deep muscles, only the larger superficial ones traverse progressively larger numbers of spinal segments.

These deepest, single-segment muscles are part of the deep layer of spinal muscles collectively called the *transversospinalis*. This term describes those muscles confined to the rope-like tenderloin of muscle that fills the laminar groove between the transverse and spinous processes on both sides up the entire spine. This includes the three muscle groups named above, as well as the rotatores longus, which likewise run from the spinous process (SP) down and out to the transverse process (TP), but cover two segments instead of just one.

The rotatores longus and rotatores brevis are assisted by the misnamed levatores costarum, which run in the same direction, down and out, from the TP to the proximal portion of the rib. Ill-positioned to 'lift the ribs' as the Latin name implies, these muscles assist the rotatores in creating twisting of the spine and ribs on each other. The levatores costarum, like the rotatores, have a brevis covering one segment, and a longus covering two segments.

The multifidus muscles present the same pattern as the rotatores – down and out from one SP to the TPs of the vertebrae three and four spinal segments below. The semispinalis repeats this pattern, but for five and six spinal segments. Though the pattern is the same, the more segments covered means that the orientation of these longer muscles is more vertical, and the action is more and more centered on extension for these outer muscles. The small ones, as their name implies, have more to do with rotation. The multifidi extend right down onto the sacral segments of the spine, securely anchoring the transversospinalis group to the pelvis.

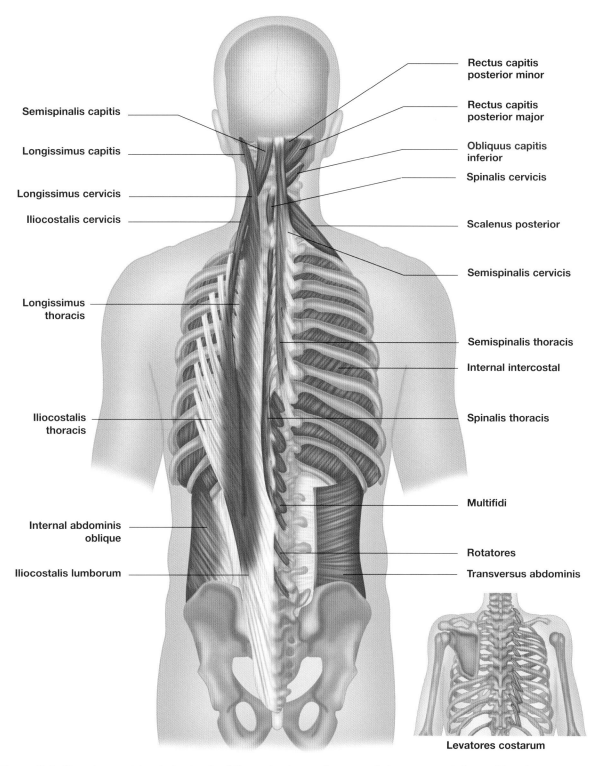

Rectus capitis posterior minor

Rectus capitis posterior major

Obliquus capitis inferior

Spinalis cervicis

Scalenus posterior

Semispinalis cervicis

Semispinalis thoracis

Internal intercostal

Spinalis thoracis

Multifidi

Rotatores

Transversus abdominis

Semispinalis capitis

Longissimus capitis

Longissimus cervicis

Iliocostalis cervicis

Longissimus thoracis

Iliocostalis thoracis

Internal abdominis oblique

Iliocostalis lumborum

Levatores costarum

Figure 8.6: The deepest (and shortest) of the spinal muscles reveal the pattern followed by the longer overlying erectors. The levatores costarum really should be called 'rotatores lateralis' or some such, as they are more active in helping the rotatores twist the spine than they are in lifting the ribs in breathing. The erector spinae are very fascial muscles with predominantly slow-twitch endurance fibers that work all day to keep us from curling up in a ball. Most medial are the spinalis and semispinalis. In the middle are the cables of the longissimus. On the outside, near the angle of the ribs, lie the small complex slips of the iliocostalis.

The Erector Spine

The outer layers of musculature are yet longer expressions of these same patterns. Taking the erector spinae from medial to lateral, the spinalis muscles (and semispinalis in the neck – more on this later) draws the spinous processes together over many segments. This small muscle – not much more than a centimeter or two wide at its most prominent part – can be found just lateral to the spinous processes. Most easily felt around T8 or so, it can then be traced up and down a few inches in either direction from there.

The longissimus complex is perhaps our hardest-working group of muscles, and can frequently be found as a set of readily palpable cables running parallel to the spine about five centimeters (two inches) either side of the spinous processes. The more 'clumpy' these cables, the less differentiated the movement of the spine. Though these muscles express the TP to SP pattern in the spine, the larger the number of segments each fascicle of the muscle crosses makes the line of pull practically vertical, and ensures that this is mostly an erector of the spine, not a rotator like its deeper counterparts.

The most lateral muscle of the spine is the iliocostalis. This runs from the posterior iliac crest progressively up the ribs just laterally to the TP, but medially to the angle of the ribs. This muscle continues the intertransversarii pattern, but in this case it is joining rib to rib rather than TP to TP. This muscle, more involved with side-bending as well as extending the spine, can usually be felt as a series of small tendons just medial to the angle of the ribs. Again, around T8 is the easiest place to palpate the muscle, which can then be traced superiorly and inferiorly from that spot. Inferiorly, the muscle mass blends with that of the longissimus in the lumbar region.

These muscles are surrounded by the various laminae of the thoracolumbar fascia. This plays a vital role in transferring the tension from the muscles evenly to the vertebrae of the lower spine and abdomen, and contralaterally, from one side of the ribs to the opposite hip, across the lumbosacral midline. This oblique load transfer is a bit independent from the muscles themselves, which run vertically, and carry many vertical tendons within themselves. These muscles contain so much fascia, in fact, that they are like the strapping tape you find at the post office: tough, fibrous and very strong. The predominance with the muscles is of slow-twitch, endurance-style muscle fibers, as these muscles must stay lightly 'on' all day and half the night, to keep us from folding up on the floor.

With all the overlying laminae of shoulder muscles, the retinacula of the serratus posterior, and the thoracolumbar fascia, as well as the strong complex of investing fascia and intramuscular tendons, these strong and thick muscles lend themselves to repeated treatment. The back work outlined in this book, along with its many variations, is designed to be applied many times, progressively opening deeper layers of these muscles to fully responsive function.

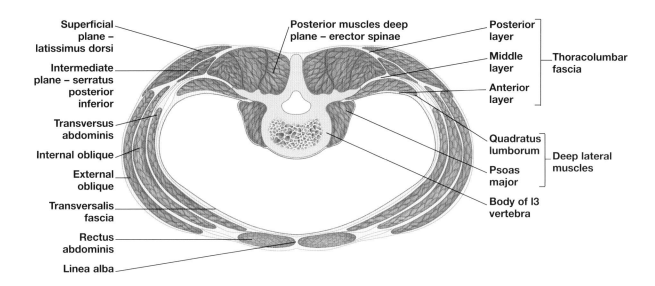

Superficial plane – latissimus dorsi

Intermediate plane – serratus posterior inferior

Transversus abdominis

Internal oblique

External oblique

Transversalis fascia

Rectus abdominis

Linea alba

Posterior muscles deep plane – erector spinae

Posterior layer

Middle layer

Anterior layer

Thoracolumbar fascia

Quadratus lumborum

Psoas major

Body of l3 vertebra

Deep lateral muscles

Figure 8.7: The erector spinae are entirely encased in the envelope of the thoracolumbar fascia, with laminae going superficial to and deep to these muscles. The serratus posterior muscles – essentially retinacula for the erectors – lie in the outer layer. Both the outer and the inner layer connect to the abdominal muscles. This fascia also transfers strain from the hips to the contralateral ribs and shoulder, and vice-versa.

The Neck

The muscle patterns we have described above continue into the neck. The neck is, however, more complicated, and requires more delicacy to deal with the smaller muscles, the many visceral tubes that pass through it, and the easily adjusted small cervical vertebrae. The neck therefore gets its own section, and the corresponding techniques should be practiced with a soft hand and attentive care.

The neck is best seen as three *cylinders* of fascia. The *outer cylinder* contains the large surrounding sheets of muscle. This contains the other two cylinders: the *visceral cylinder* in the front and the *motor cylinder* surrounding the vertebrae behind it in back. Gently pinch your larynx and move it left and right to see how easily moveable the visceral cylinder is within the body. Reaching around to the back of your neck and trying to move the motor cylinder in a similar way will show how tight and self-regulating the motor cylinder is, as opposed to the 'passive' visceral cylinder.

Our discussion of the neck is devoted to the superficial cylinder and the complex motor cylinder. The visceral cylinder muscles, consisting of the hyoid complex and the related muscles under the tongue, are left for a later volume.

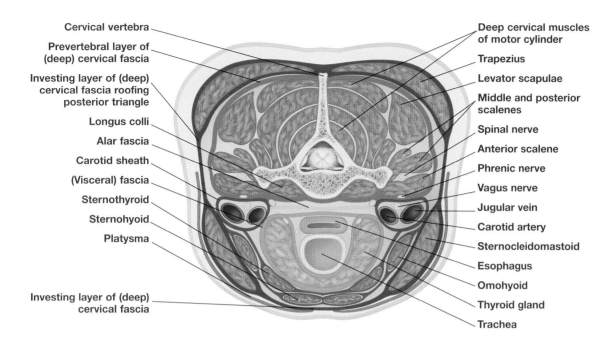

Cervical vertebra
Prevertebral layer of (deep) cervical fascia
Investing layer of (deep) cervical fascia roofing posterior triangle
Longus colli
Alar fascia
Carotid sheath
(Visceral) fascia
Sternothyroid
Sternohyoid
Platysma
Investing layer of (deep) cervical fascia

Deep cervical muscles of motor cylinder
Trapezius
Levator scapulae
Middle and posterior scalenes
Spinal nerve
Anterior scalene
Phrenic nerve
Vagus nerve
Jugular vein
Carotid artery
Sternocleidomastoid
Esophagus
Omohyoid
Thyroid gland
Trachea

Figure 8.8: The fascia of the neck essentially consists of three cylinders: a superficial one around the whole neck, containing an anterior 'visceral cylinder' and a posterior 'motor cylinder' which surrounds the cervical vertebrae with a protecting and motivating complex.

The Superficial Cylinder: Trapezius and Sternocleidomastoid

Although one can find the platysma in the skin of the neck (the 'yikes' muscle that makes the skin between the chin and chest stand out), the primary protectors and movers of the neck lie in the bilaminar layer of the fascia colli superficialis. Beginning at the spinous processes and the ligamentum nuchae, the trapezius – tucked within this fascia – wraps around the posterior neck. The trapezius is of course a shoulder muscle, dealt with in Chapter 9 in terms of its relation to the arm, but it also functions to protect and turn the neck.

The very topmost portion of the trapezius is the occipito-clavicular part – running from the posteromedial aspect of the occiput down and forward to the lateral third of the clavicle. The next section down of the trapezius – the cervico-acromial portion – runs from the cervical SPs down and out to the tip of the shoulder-blade. Both these parts are contralateral rotators (like the sternocleidomastoid) of the head on the shoulders, and also elevators of the shoulder. Sometimes their function, however, runs in the other direction (we would call this *dysfunction*), and the shoulder becomes involved in steadying the neck and head. This common functional fault involves the appendicular shoulder in the axial function of head stability, and paves the way for many a shoulder injury.

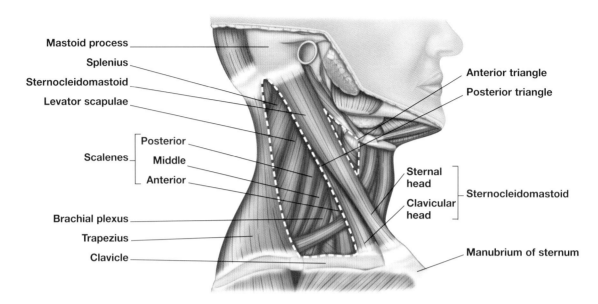

Figure 8.9: The sternocleidomastoid and trapezius start life as the same muscle – it is the growth of the collarbone that separates them. This creates a long, thin triangle between the two, a fascial window through which we can reach the motor cylinder. Sometimes the trapezius is called upon to dysfunctionally substitute for the SCM.

The sternocleidomastoid (SCM) covers the side and front of the neck. The SCM is a contralateral rotator of the head, but often has more function as a postural muscle that in dysfunction helps to pull the head down and forward. The SCM and trapezius are invested in the same fascial casing. The direction this fascia needs to be moved in almost everyone is up and back, to counter the downward and forward drag.

These two muscles start out, in fact, as one in the embryo, and are split into two by the growth of the collarbone. The lower attachments of the two-headed SCM are the easily palpable head that goes to the sternum, and the wider and more lateral head that goes to the medial third of the clavicle.

Thus the leading edge of the trapezius and the trailing edge of the SCM are separated by the middle third of the clavicle at the bottom. At their top, at the lateral occiput and posterior temporal bones, the two muscles are closely adjacent and their fasciae blend with each other (as well as going up onto the skull to blend with the epicranial fascia). The long, thin oblique triangle thus created between the two is a 'window' into the scalenes and other muscles of the motor cylinder deep to this encircling superficial sleeve.

The Motor Cylinder

The motor cylinder consists of the thirteen or so muscles that attach around the stacked tower of the cervical vertebrae, mainly to the transverse processes. These could be grouped as (1) the longus muscles in the front, (2) the scalenes and levator scapulae to the side, and (3) the splenius muscles, enclosing the spinal muscles in back.

Taking these in turn, the longus colli and longus capitis run up the front of the neck. When they shorten they flex the neck, or, just as importantly, they prevent hyperextension. Thus these muscles need to be toned in the case of a hyperextended cervical curve (cervical lordosis, common in many a head-forward posture), or lengthened in the case of reduced or reverse curvature (military neck).

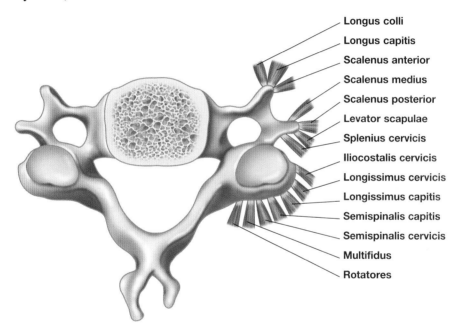

Longus colli
Longus capitis
Scalenus anterior
Scalenus medius
Scalenus posterior
Levator scapulae
Splenius cervicis
Iliocostalis cervicis
Longissimus cervicis
Longissimus capitis
Semispinalis capitis
Semispinalis cervicis
Multifidus
Rotatores

Figure 8.10: Many muscles compete for space in attaching to (principally) the transverse processes of the cervical vertebrae. These include (1) longus colli, (2) longus capitis, (3) anterior scalene (note the gully posterior to this muscle for the brachial nerves), (4) middle scalene, (5) posterior scalene, (6) levator scapulae, (7) splenius cervicis wrapping around, (8) iliocostalis, (9) longissimus, (10) semispinalis, (11) multifidus, and finally (12) rotatores.

Find these muscles carefully by lying your client on their back, with you sitting at the head end of the table. Leaning in so your elbows are wide and your fingers are aiming for each other, put your fingertips palms down, under the trailing edge of the SCM, and lift the SCM with the fingernail side of your digits. You will feel, deep to the SCM, the hard myofascial trunk of the motor cylinder, specifically the scalenes. Let your fingertips slide into the space in front of the scalenes, between the motor and the visceral cylinder. In this way, you allow all the visceral concerns in the visceral cylinder to be safe. Desist if any of this causes brachial plexus stimulation, or if your client turns beetroot red in the face.

If you keep your elbows wide and slide directly in front of the scalenes, you will be able to feel the bumps of the transverse processes (TPs) under your finger pads. The longus colli (which reaches all the way down into the chest to the front of T4) and longus capitis will be just medial to these TPs, and will pop into your fingers at the slightest suggestion of lifting the head. In the case of postural hyperextension, your fingers' presence is only to help the client find her longus muscles and to activate them. If they are short and the neck has a reduced or reverse curvature, then you can use your fingers here as tools to lengthen them.

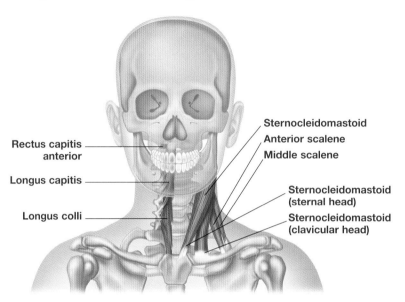

Figure 8.11: The longus muscles, running along the front of the neck, must be engaged to keep the neck from collapsing into hyperextension, but must be released if the neck is stuck in flexion. The middle and posterior scalenes both limit and create side-to-side movement of the neck. The anterior scalene between is unique in either lifting the upper rib in the breath, or (in dysfunction) pulling the lower neck vertebrae down and forward instead.

Lateral to the TPs is the 'skirt' of the three scalene muscles. The brachial plexus (and the brachial artery) emerges between the anterior and the middle scalene, so palpate with delicacy and caution. That said, the scalenes provide major lateral support for the neck, and these muscles themselves are tough and highly fascial.

For the anterior scalene, position your hands again at the posterior edge of SCM, near the collarbone. Again, lift the SCM up with the fingernails, and slide the fingertips under the clavicular head. The anterior scalene is a dense band, about one and a half centimeters (one-half inch) wide, just deep to the clavicular head of the SCM. It will activate during the inhalation phase of breathing, sometimes all the way through the breath, sometimes only near the top of the breath. This muscle – or, more correctly, *myofascial complex* – is designed to pull up on the upper two ribs in breathing. Unfortunately, its up and backward pull on the ribs is converted instead, when the ribs are more fixed, into a down and forward pull on the lower cervical vertebrae. Use the techniques in this book to restore proper function to the lower neck and upper ribs.

The middle and posterior scalenes are incompletely separate muscles, so they get treated together. These two operate together as the 'quadratus lumborum' of the neck, preventing too much side-to-side movement of the head. The fascia from these muscles also reaches into the shoulder, and can be implicated when the shoulders are at different levels.

You can find the middle scalene easily: it is the most lateral muscle of the motor cylinder, and can be felt as the most prominent muscle (deep to the SCM and trapezius) when you 'strum' the side of the neck like a guitar; it feels like a distinct and prominent string on that guitar. The posterior scalene lies behind and just medial to the middle scalene, so tucking a fingertip in behind the middle picks up its helpmate, the posterior scalene.

The levator scapulae is easily found just behind the posterior scalene. Place three fingertips somewhere just behind the scalenes, reach across with your other hand and hold the shoulder blade down. Ask your client to lift their shoulder-blade against the resistance of your hand, and the levator scapulae will pop into your fingers. Once it does, it can be followed under the trapezius to the apex of the scapula, or up to the TPs just posterior to the scalene attachments.

Posterior to the levator scapulae, the splenius muscles – capitis and cervicis – wrap around the spinal muscles we have previously detailed (see page 189). The iliocostalis is the most lateral, reaching up into the neck, but not as far as the head. The longissimus does have a connection all the way to the skull, attaching deep to the mastoid process underneath the SCM and digastric. The semispinalis and multifidus muscles, bound together in the vertical cord, can be strummed about two and one-half centimeters (one inch) from the spinous process in the middle of the back of the neck. This major anchor for the head is put under strain (eccentric loading) in head-forward posture.

At the very deepest level lie the suboccipitals, a group of small but very important muscles. These are the rectus capitis posterior minor (RCPM), rectus capitis posterior major (RCPMaj), obliquus capitis superior (OCS) and obliquus capitis inferior (OCI). Two other muscles in this group, rectus capitis lateralis and rectus capitis anterior, are difficult to find and treat, and will be left for a future volume.

These muscles form a star, based around the prominent spinous process of the second cervical vertebra (the axis), which can be easily felt as the first available SP below the occiput, the atlas having virtually no spinous process at all. If you insinuate your thumbs under your occiput just to either side of this SP, with your fingers on the side of your head to keep it from moving, and roll your eyes in a circle (open or closed, it does not matter), you will feel the tonus of these muscles change under your thumbs. These muscles have a high number of muscle spindles, and they are hard-wired to your eyes. As your eyes move, these muscles 'listen' to that movement, and adjust the spine accordingly. This is the mechanism a cat uses to land on its feet, straightening the spine super-fast after it locates the horizontal with its eyes and inner ear.

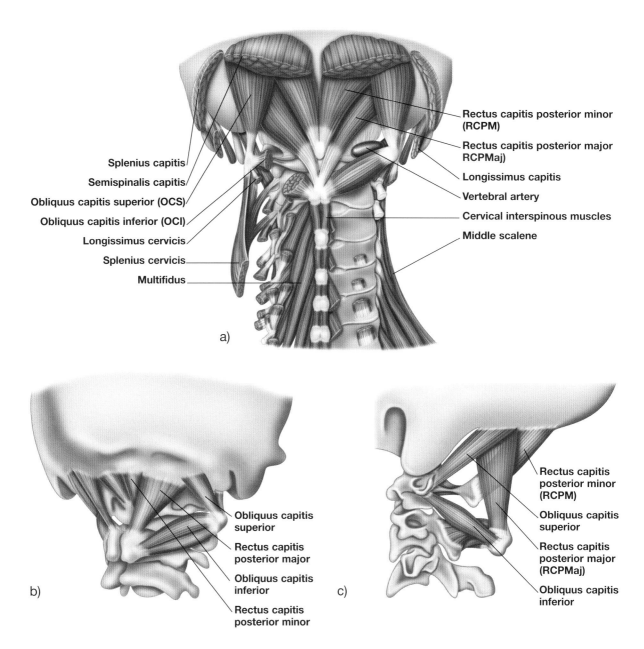

Splenius capitis
Semispinalis capitis
Obliquus capitis superior (OCS)
Obliquus capitis inferior (OCI)
Longissimus cervicis
Splenius cervicis
Multifidus

Rectus capitis posterior minor (RCPM)
Rectus capitis posterior major RCPMaj)
Longissimus capitis
Vertebral artery
Cervical interspinous muscles
Middle scalene

a)

Obliquus capitis superior
Rectus capitis posterior major
Obliquus capitis inferior
Rectus capitis posterior minor

b)

Rectus capitis posterior minor (RCPM)
Obliquus capitis superior
Rectus capitis posterior major (RCPMaj)
Obliquus capitis inferior

c)

Figure 8.12: In (a), we see this suboccipital group from the back, a view presented in all anatomies. An oblique view (b) shows how the muscles run in different directions to create different moments of rotation. In (c), we can see how the RCPM and OCS pull down and forward on the occiput in such a way as to pull the occiput in toward the atlas – an aberration that shows up often in fear patterns, myopia and post-traumatic situations.

Retraction of these muscles produces a forward movement of the occiput on the atlas, and takes the head into hyperextension. Such retraction is a very common fear response, and will frequently be found in the anxious patient. Unilateral shortness in the OCS produces postural rotation of the skull on the neck. Unilateral shortness in the OCI is very common, as it always accompanies a rotation in the spine, which needs to be compensated for in the atlanto-axial joint, leading to one-sided tension in the OCI.

To find the OCI, put your fingertip in the 'divot' just behind and below the mastoid process, in between the top of the SCM and the top of the trapezius. Go toward the center of the neck at about forty-five degrees, through the splenius and the underlying multifidus, to the OCI. Put your thumbs or palms on the client's head and have them turn one way and then the other against your resistance. You will feel the OCI contract on the side to which they are turning. You will also feel the difference (if any, but it is very common) between the standing tonus on each side.

The other three muscles – RCPM, RCPMaj and OCS – can be felt deep along the back of the occiput. Sitting at your supine client's head, slide your hands under the skull, so that the occiput is resting comfortably in the curve of your palm, and your fingers are free down the neck. Flex your fingers, bringing six fingertips – the second through fourth on each hand (leave the little fingers extended on the table) – onto the bottom of the occiput. To be properly positioned, your ring fingers should be almost touching in the middle, just at the nuchal ligament, and your index fingertips should still be on the back of the occiput (not around to the side with the mastoid process). Your fingertips should be pointing back toward you, not toward the ceiling. They should be as far under the occiput as you can manage, as if to hook the occiput and bring it toward you up the table.

In this position, the RCPMaj will lie under your middle fingertip (and can usually be felt as a distinct string or mound if you strum back and forth with this finger). The other two muscles, RCPM and OCS – starting deep and going down and forward from there – cannot usually be distinctly felt. If the middle finger is on RCPMaj, however, then the other two fingertips will automatically position themselves properly.

It is difficult to overestimate the effect that release of these muscles can have on the movement in the spine, release of the sacrum, diminution of headaches, release of vision, correction of head-forward posture, relaxation of the fear response and plain old neck and head mobility. These muscles are the functional centerpiece of the Superficial Back Line, and a focus of the Alexander Technique.

The spinal armature floats within this sea of large and small soft tissue components. The complexity of the spine commands respect, care and years of careful study, but we should not be afraid to work in the soft tissue that works the spine, as here we find release for many deep patterns.

BodyReading the Spine

The spine is a wonderful piece of biological engineering surrounded by a series of supporting cables we call muscles (but that are actually myofascia), allowing movement through a wide range. It is one of the most common reasons for people turning up at our doorstep. Our aim is to help re-create natural, balanced curves, to reduce any side-to-side bends, and finally to re-align the rotations. Our work will progress in that order, starting with front to back issues, then side-to-side bends or tilts, followed by resolving any rotations. As it can be a little complicated, we have taken a couple of case histories to work our way through the examples.

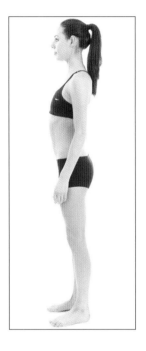

Figure 8.13: Reading the curves of the spine. When we look at our model, we can see the long posterior bend in her lumbar vertebrae, extending all the way up to her mid/upper thoracic vertebrae. The anterior shift of her head is then achieved by quite a sharp anterior bend in the upper thoracic vertebrae and lower cervical vertebrae.

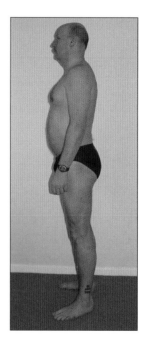

Figure 8.14: This model demonstrates a similar posterior bend in the lumbar vertebrae, but it is then followed by a long anterior bend from the mid-thoracic into the lower cervical area.

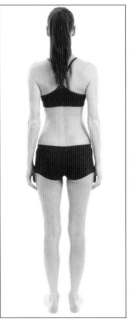

Figure 8.15: The back view will reveal lateral tilts and bends in the spine. Here we see a tilt to the left in the lumbar vertebrae, which is slowly corrected by a bend to the right (obscured here by the ponytail) in the upper thoracics. The latter is unfortunately obscured by the hair of the ponytail.

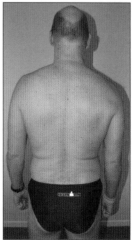

Figure 8.16: This close-up shows quite a long and strong bend of the spine from approximately T12 to T3, after which the spine bends back to the left in the lower neck to achieve a more vertical head position.

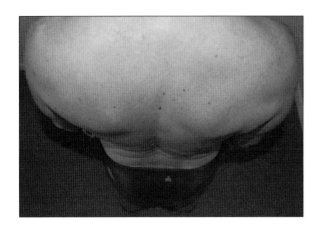
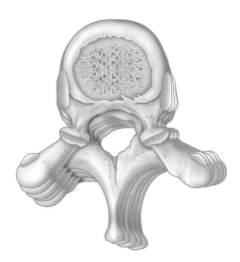

Figure 8.17a & b: By looking straight down the model's back, we can see that the erectors on the right are more posterior than the left in the mid- to lower thoracic area. Unless the client is doing strongly one-sided exercise or movement, this can be taken as a reasonable indicator of the spinal positions whereby the gradual rotation of the vertebra causes the transverse processes on the right, in this case, to push the erectors posteriorly, as shown in figure 8.17b.

Spine Techniques

Erector Spinae – Back Stripes (SBL)

The erectors will of course be involved in all the many different spinal and thorax positions, but the first plane on which we try to balance them is the sagittal, to deal with the differing degrees of flexion and extension, and to balance the primary and secondary curves of the spine.

When the spine flexes and the erectors are fascially restricted, the tendency is for the erectors to migrate laterally away from the spinous processes. The reverse occurs when the spine is held in relative postural extension: the erectors myofascia moves medially toward the spinous processes.

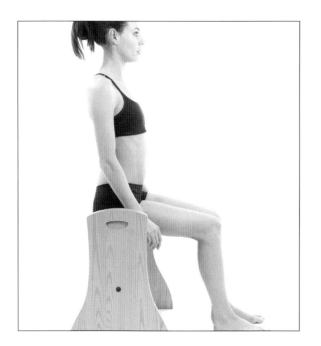

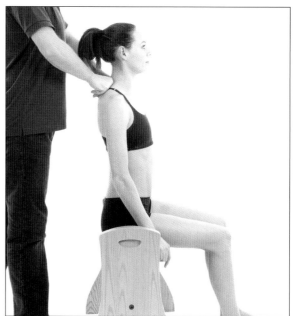

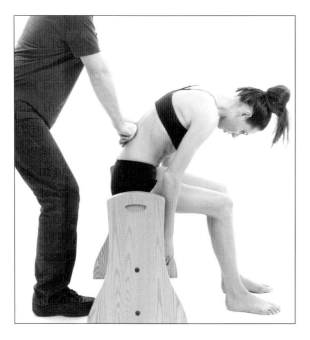

Figure 8.18 (a & b): After seating the client correctly, have them slowly roll forward (c), one vertebra at a time, as you draw the erector spinae tissue inferiorly. Each repetition of the stroke can be a little deeper, working progressively into the bellies of the erectors.

Experience this yourself by flexing your thoracic spine as you are reading this and then extend to straighten up again. Feel how the tissue across the back spreads as you flex and draws medially as you extend. Whilst other myofascial elements will also need to be corrected, it is useful, and sometimes efficacious on its own, to bring the erector tissue back to its more natural resting place.

To prepare the tissue and to help balance the front/back fascial planes, start with simple back stripes. Seat the client on a bench or suitable stool, hips slightly higher than their knees – certainly not lower – and feet roughly hip-width apart and in front of their knees. Coach your client in the correct procedure to roll forward, one vertebra at a time, the top of their head going out and over their knees, in order not to collapse into their abdomen.

Let them practice this once or twice while you get a visual or palpatory assessment of any restricted sections in the spine, where the spinous processes do not fan away from each other. Then place your knuckles of the index and ring fingers glide down the tissue either side of the spine in concert with the client's movement. The intention is to open the tissue around the erectors, drawing the deep investing fascia inferiorly and preparing the tissue for more specific work.

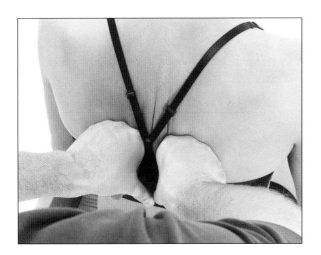
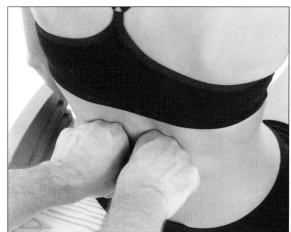
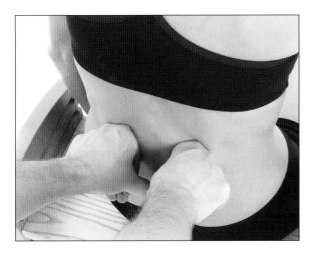

Figure 8.19a, b & c: To help correct the medial or lateral migration of the erectors and their associated tissue, the tissue can be drawn medially (a) or laterally (b & c).

After warming and preparing the tissue, the next stage is to work with the migration of the tissue. If it has moved laterally because of too much flexion (or anterior bend) in the spine, then draw it medially. If it is attaching too medially, then try to bring it away from the spinous processes. In Rachael's case she needs only the upper thoracic erectors brought medially (please note for visual clarity the technique is shown at a lower level) and then, because of her long posterior bend, the rest of the erector tissue can be brought laterally.

Erector Spinae – Spinal Bends (SBL)

When the spine bends to one side it creates a shortness (or is caused by that shortness!) of the erector spinae on the side to which it bends. If we look again at the bends of the spine of both models in figures 8.15 and 8.16, we can see that the right erectors in the mid-thoracic region are shorter and also further away from the spine. The erectors on the left must therefore be longer and closer to the spinous processes. If we are to help correct this pattern, then we need to remodel the fascial connections by reversing this relationship. We do this by bringing the lateral tissue medially and the more medial tissue laterally.

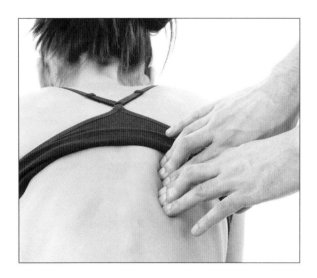

Figure 8.20: With your client seated on the bench, have them lean forward, supporting their elbows on their knees, and engage the tissue lateral to the short erectors.

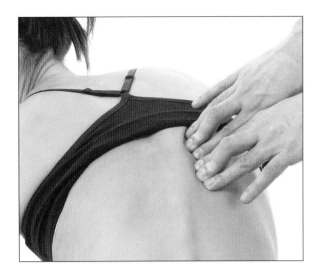

Figure 8.21: Have the client then bend to the opposite side as you encourage the tissue to move medially.

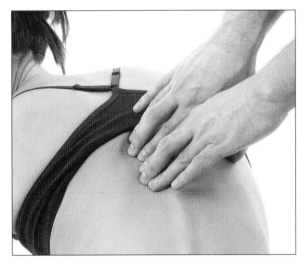

Figure 8.22: Release and re-engage on the other side of the spine, this time medial to the erector spinae tissue, and tease the muscles laterally as the client again bends to the opposite side.

This technique could also be done with the client prone on the table, reaching down along one side of their body to lengthen the opposite side, as you work with the tissue in the same way as above. This prone technique is fine for initially opening tissue, but the best integration of the new position and movement will come with the bench work; so it is best to finish up with this bench work after doing any prone table work.

Spinal Rotations

Different portions of the spine have differing abilities to rotate, depending on the nature of the vertebral joints, as described above. Those of you who are keen to take this rewarding area of work further are encouraged to read and study further; there are many worthy references given in the bibliography. We need to be clear that we are not adjusting or manipulating the spine in the way of physiotherapy, osteopathy or chiropractic, but simply using the soft tissue as the elastics in the spinal tensegrity to ease both interosseous relationship and intraosseous strain.

We also want to point out and remind ourselves that we read the body according to itself and not in accordance with anybody's particular rules of spinal mechanics. In our experience, the body often varies from these laws, taking its own course through life in ignorance of the tenets it *should* be following. Treat each spine in its glorious individuality. The rotations of the spine will be held by the deep spinal muscles, that last deep layer of the plywood arrangement of tissue on the back. These short oblique muscles will pull the spinous processes toward one of the transverse processes of the vertebra below, tending to turn the spine to the opposite side.

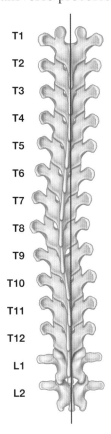

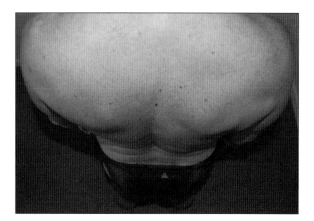

Figure 8.23a & b: If we look again down our model's back, we can see the rotation begin around L2 and continue until approximately T3, where the spine and erectors seem to lose any rotation. In order to come from neutral and back again the spine will have to rotate in both directions. In (b), we see how the rotation reaches an apex at T8 with its spinous process the most deviated from midline and then each subsequent vertebra above it moves gradually back toward the midline.

In the model's case above, with his rotation to the right we can see that there is a progression in the rotation (can you separate this from the larger, more evident bend?). It begins in the upper lumbar vertebrae and reaches its peak at around T7/T8, before correcting gradually. This means that the spinal segments are rotated to the right between L1/L2 and T7/T8; but then, as the rotation corrects itself, it must be rotating back to the left between T7/T8 and T2/T3.

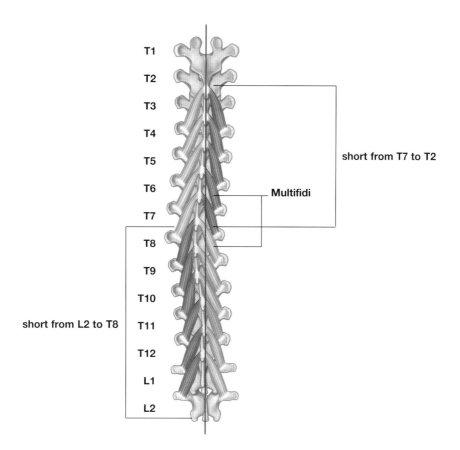

T1
T2
T3
T4
T5
T6
T7
T8
T9
T10
T11
T12
L1
L2

short from T7 to T2

Multifidi

short from L2 to T8

Figure 8.24: For clarity the multifidi have been represented as single joint muscles only to show how the spinal rotators are short on the left until the level of T8, after which point they rotate in the other direction and are therefore shortened on the opposite side.

If we carry on with this case history, the spinous processes of L1 are connected to the transverse processes of the vertebrae two, three and four segments lower. So in order to adjust these guy ropes, we must commence our stroke at that level, four segments below the start of the rotation. We would continue in the same manner, starting the stroke four segments below and releasing the tissue up and in toward the spinous process in question.

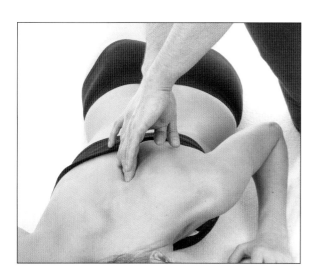

Figure: 8.25: Standing to the side with the short multifidi, sink your fingers into the deep spinal muscles, entering via the palpable 'valley' between the spinous process and the erector spinae. Have your client place their hand under the shoulder on the same side and ask them to push into it to turn the section in the opposite direction of their rotation. As the client turns, lengthen the multifidi by taking the tissue medially and superiorly, taking care not to press onto the spinous process.

So we would repeat the stroke up to the point at which the rotation starts to correct itself and, as we saw earlier, this is where the vertebrae are rotated in the other direction relative to each other. Our last stroke to correct the right rotation will approach T7 from the left side in this example. We then need to swap onto the other side of the client to approach T6 from four spinal segments below to correct the compensatory left rotation (figure 8.26a & b).

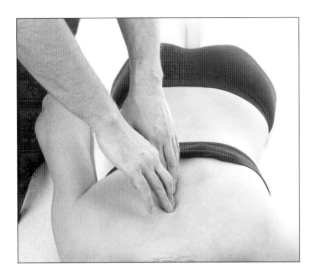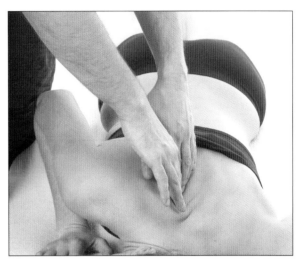

Figure 8.26a & b: Starting four segments below the beginning of the rotation, engage the deep spinal rotators and lengthen them toward the spinous process of the left-rotated vertebra, as the client de-rotates herself to the side on which you are working from by pushing the torso into a rotation with her hand.

As with the side-bends, this work can be done on the bench, but the overall technique remains the same. By using their own hands on either side of their trunk, the client can lock certain areas to restrict the rotation, in order to focus it at other levels.

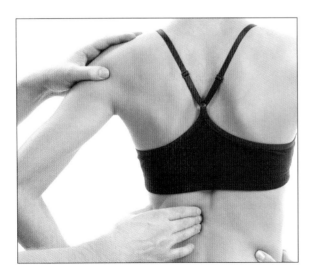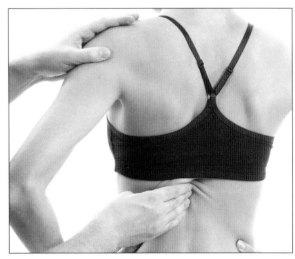

Figure 8.27a & b: Kneeling to one side of the client, use your fingers in exactly the same fashion as with the prone method, drawing tissue up and in as the client rotates. This position can be particularly useful for thoracic rotations as the rhomboids and trapezius can remain relaxed.

Side-Lying Thoracolumbar Fascia (BFL, SFAL and SBL)

The thoracolumbar fascia plays an important role in the stability of the low back, and much research has been done into its many roles. Freedom from restriction can be vital in the restoration of a healthy back.

You can either sit on the couch to use the fingertips of the working hand, or stand to use a soft fist created by the same hand. Engage the thick, often restricted tissue over the lumbar and sacral areas in a superior direction and ask the client to slowly tilt their pelvis posteriorly ('tuck their tail under'). Take a number of different sections to cover the areas thoroughly. The effectiveness of the stretch created by the client's movement will be strongest closer to the apex of the sacrum and will diminish as you travel superiorly. Just feel for when the returns no longer justify the extra work you need to put in.

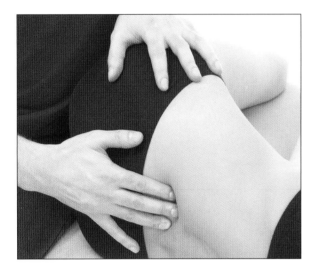 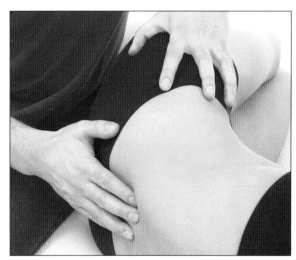

Figure 8.28a & b: Keep your fingers straight (or substitute a soft fist) and use your non-working hand to guide the client's pelvis and the client's timing as they 'tuck their tail under'.

The client will be re-educating many muscles, so there are many secondary benefits in this technique for strengthening, coordinating and bringing awareness to the many muscles surrounding and controlling the pelvis. The technique can also be used to introduce many core stability type lessons; for example, by having the client engage their transversus abdominis as they do the movement.

This can be hard work for your fingers initially, so maybe start with just using your fingers to engage over the sacrum and then change to a fist for the lower back.

Side-Lying Quadratus Lumborum (LTL and DFL)

Quadratus lumborum (QL) muscle is involved in most back pain issues. Because its fascia spans the gap between the ilium and the twelfth rib and attaches to each of the lumbar vertebrae, it will be greatly affected by – and affect the position of – all three bony regions.

Familiarize yourself with the alignment of the three different layers of QL and you will see that there are varying directions of force it can produce. The vertical fibers will be more involved with spinal extension or side flexion, but the angled fibers will either pull the lumbar vertebrae toward the ilium (lower, iliolumbar fibers) or pull the twelfth rib toward the lumbar vertebrae (upper, lumbocostal fibers). This will be important when dealing with lateral shifts of the thorax relative to the pelvis, the kind of pattern one would see in parents who carry their child on one hip to leave the dominant hand free for various tasks. Mimic this pattern on yourself and feel what happens to the lumbar vertebrae of one side and the twelfth rib on the other. If you shift your rib cage to the left, can you feel how the lumbar vertebrae have moved closer to the left ilium but your right twelfth rib has moved down, closer to your lumbar vertebrae on the right?

The type of work performed on the fascia around the QL will differ greatly, depending on the client's postural pattern. In a flatback or military-type posture it will need to be brought toward the midline rather than lengthened, but for an anteriorly tilted pelvis or posteriorly tilted thorax it will require opening in this area to help ease any increase in the lordotic curve of the lumbar vertebrae.

To find the QL fascia, fold your fingertips over the lip of the ilium and, starting roughly along the midline, walk posteriorly. Without moving too far you should feel an 'edge' in the deeper tissue; this should be the lateral aspect of the QL fascia. Orient your finger along the edge and engage into the tissue with a hook superiorly. Ask the client to slowly lengthen their upper leg toward the bottom of the couch. A more movement-aware client may be able to achieve the same effect by simply tilting their pelvis, dropping their ischial tuberosity away from their ribs.

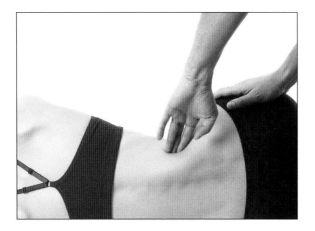 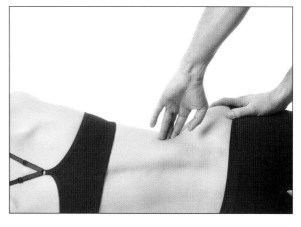

Figure 8.29a & b: Engaging the tissue toward the head will help release the inferior portion of the QL, as the client reaches away with the upper leg.

With the hook in the superior direction, you will isolate the stretch in the lower portion of the tissue, the iliolumbar fibers. In order to open the upper, lumbocostal fibers, angle your engagement inferiorly. With the same movement from the client, you will assist the stretch by both working in the same direction but challenging the superior aspect of the QL.

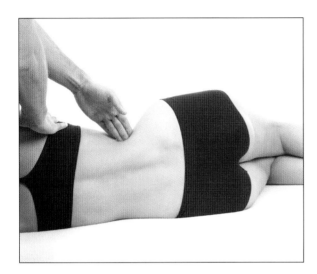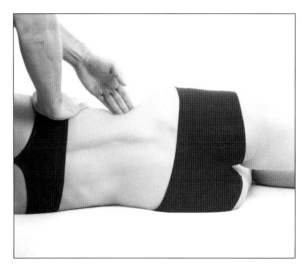

Figure 8.30a & b: Using a caudal direction will help isolate the release into the upper fibers of QL. The non-working hand can be used to guide the pelvis and/or to help increase the stretch. It is shown resting on the rib cage and could act as a cue to draw the breath into the lateral ribs, which will also help increase the stretch.

It can be important to isolate both aspects when trying to lengthen the whole of the lumbar area, and so working in both directions on both sides will achieve better results. In lateral shifts of the rib cage on the pelvis, best results will be obtained by working differently on the two sides.

Seated Quadratus Lumborum (LTL and DFL)

It can often be more educational, and more effective, to have the client seated on a bench for low back work. Ensure the bench you are using is of the correct height to maintain the client's engagement with the floor through their feet, with their knees just slightly lower than their hips. (Do not do this off the edge of a high massage couch with the client's feet in the air, or the result will be shortened hip flexors.) Do not use a chair or stool on wheels, and obviously find a surface that will allow both ischial tuberosities to be level.

With your elbows wide use either your fingers or knuckles to engage the lateral aspect of the QL and engage the tissue inferiorly, i.e. toward the ilium and hooking posteriorly slightly. Ask the client to slowly side-bend and maybe rotate slightly as you maintain the lock in the fascia.

This is a strong technique and may require both arm and hand strength. Remember to keep your arms wide to engage your chest muscles. Use only small movements from your client as you build the strength and sensitivity to remain engaged in the correct area.

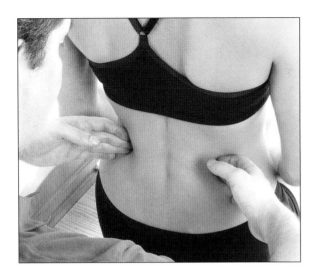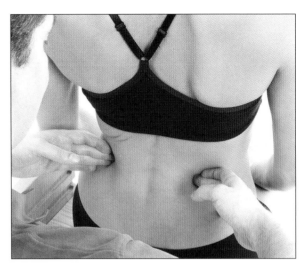

Figure 8.31a & b: Find the fascial edge of the QL on both sides, and locking into one side have the client side flex and maybe use some rotation also to open the tissue. The tissue is engaged inferiorly, and the photographs show the right side being released.

This is perhaps a more effective method of isolating the stretch into the upper fibers of the QL, as you can resist the movement more efficiently. The lower portion of QL is usually most challenged with the client in side-lying, as above.

Psoas Balancing (DFL)

The psoas major can be involved in quite a number of patterns involving the position of both the pelvis and the thorax. Since this is a triangular muscle, the medial, lower fibers can help create and maintain an increased lordotic curve, whilst the upper, lateral fibers can decrease the normal curve, helping to create a flatback pattern. Unilateral shortness can cause the thorax to tilt to that side, and perhaps eventually rotate away from it.

To work on one side at a time, sink your fingers into the abdomen medially to the ASIS. Remember to draw a little skin and adipose laterally before you start, in order not to stretch this superficial tissue as you sink into the iliac fossa. As you travel deep, follow the contour of the anterior surface of the ilium and it will guide you deep and eventually medially.

Finding the psoas major in this way can also help you assess the relationship between the psoas major and the iliacus, as they can sometimes become adhered via the iliac fascia. In these cases it is useful to spend time differentiating them by 'swimming' your fingers into the septum to tease them apart.

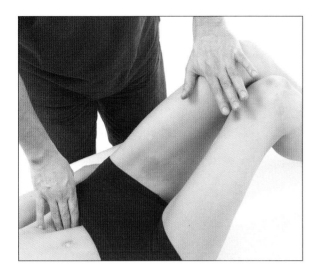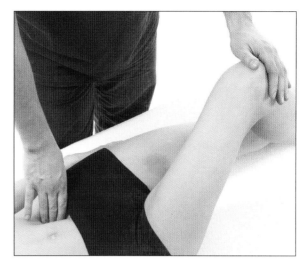

Figure 8.32a & b: The psoas major can be worked as described in Chapter 6, page 152, dealing with the thigh and pelvis.

You can then focus on the psoas major tissue. To confirm that you have found it, ask your client to lift their foot from the table. You should feel the muscle contract under your fingers. If you do not feel it directly, you may need to move a little more medially. Once you are in contact, the client may report being unable to perform the movement. This can be an indication of a weak muscle where your pressure is inhibiting it.

The lateral fibers are the ones you are more likely to engage first. If you need to access the medial fibers, keep in contact with the bulk of the muscle as you roll over it to engage the lower fibers. This will help move any fragile vessels out of the way before you press more firmly into the muscle. In either case, you can simply draw the tissue slightly superiorly and ask your client to slowly glide their heel along the table to extend their hip as you resist the lengthening of the appropriate fibers.

To work bilaterally, use both hands and find the psoas major on both sides using the same guidelines as above, and making sure your pressure is the same from both hands. Ask your client to slowly push into their feet and roll their sacrum and lumbar vertebrae up. Then engage the psoas myofascia lightly as they roll back down, one vertebra at a time. Use the input from both hands to guide the lengthening of the tissue, to ensure it is even.

When working with the psoas major ask your client to inform you if they feel any discomfort such as hot, gassy or searing pain. You may inadvertently impinge some intestinal tissue on your way to the psoas major and simply releasing and using a slightly different angle can free it again. Be aware of appendectomies and other abdominal surgeries, acting accordingly if any are present by avoiding the area, working superficially first to free any scar tissue or just paying more attention as you enter.

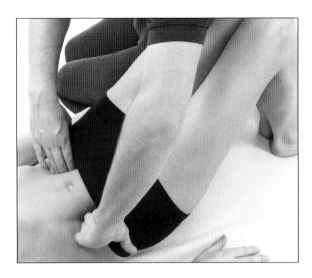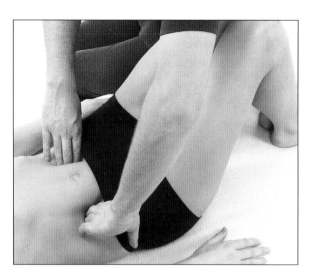

Figure 8.33a & b: Have the client roll their pelvis up by pushing into their feet. Engage the psoas major on both sides, and then monitor the lengthening of the tissue as the client rolls each vertebra back down onto the table.

BodyReading the Head and Neck

With an ideal head position, its center of gravity would be above that of the thorax. This would allow all of the supportive guy wires to do their designed tasks, without burdening them with the extra job of keeping the head cantilevered out front. Many references recommend the ear and the head of the humerus to be vertically aligned. This can lead to confusion, however, because of the independent mobility of the shoulder girdle. The shoulder girdle is in the best case not involved in stabilizing the head and neck.

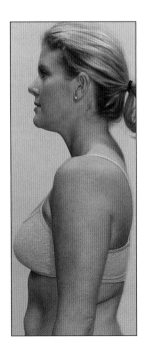

In our example (figure 8.34), the shoulders are drawn back (posteriorly shifted) to help counterbalance the head going forward. The head of the humerus is then brought anteriorly by the medial rotation of the scapula. It also appears slightly anterior within the glenohumeral joint.

We can see how all of the tissue traveling in an anterior-inferior to posterior-superior direction will be shortened (SCM, anterior portion of upper trapezius, anterior scalene and RCPM and obliquus capitis superior), while the reverse will be true of the front of the upper throat and around the cervico-thoracic junction. In this case we can see how the line of the SCM has become almost vertical, rather than angling back and up to the mastoid process.

Figure 8.34: This client clearly displays an anterior head position relative to the thorax, but her ear and the head of the humerus are not so far out of alignment if we use a plumb line.

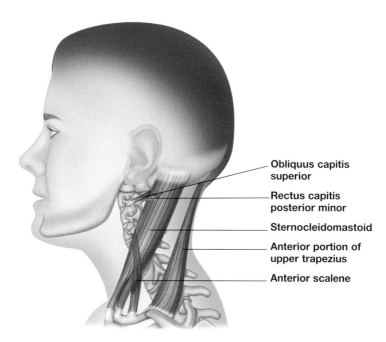

Figure 8.35: Here we can more clearly see the soft tissues that will be shortened by an anterior shift of the head.

When we see side tilts of the neck, then we are drawn particularly to the middle and posterior scalenes on the shorter side – but we must first also address the more superficial tissue of the ipsilateral trapezius and splenius cervicis. In these cases the head often corrects itself by tilting in the opposite direction from the neck to help keep the eyes oriented to the horizon. To correct this pattern we will need to include work to lengthen the suboccipitals and splenius capitis on this side.

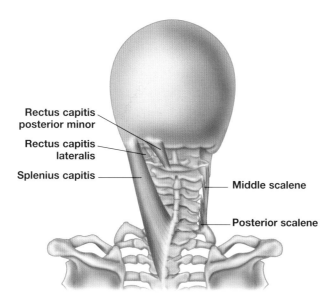

Figure 8.36: For side-to-side tilts we can see another 'X' pattern develop, matching the shortened and lengthened tissue either side of the midline.

Neck Techniques

Sternocleidomastoid (SFL and LTL)

Largest of the group of muscles that will conspire to draw the head and neck forward and downward into an anterior shift, the sternocleidomastoid (SCM) is an important guy wire for the head. Because of its proximity to the jugular vein and carotid artery, many therapists are nervous of approaching it. And justifiably so – these structures are delicate and vital, so great care must be taken. But the SCM overlying them often requires lengthening as an important first step in getting balance around the highly mobile head and neck.

This first stroke is designed to open the fascia surrounding the muscle, drawing it posteriorly in the process. Start by standing on the side to be worked and ask your client to turn their head as if it was turning on a pole, or as if they had a lollipop stick through the middle of their head (use your own image or the one that makes sense of the movement to the client). Their movement can also be guided by using your upper hand on the top of the head, with the fingers spread to encourage the client to keep their head in contact with the same part of the couch as they turn – quite a different movement from rolling the head along the table.

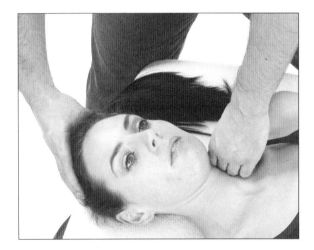
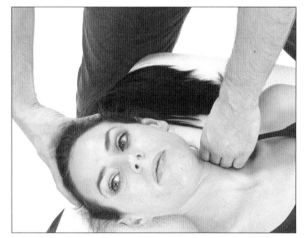

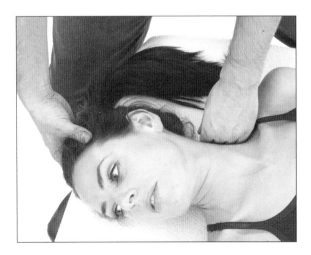

Figure 8.37a, b & c: Ensuring your engagement remains at the level of the SCM and anterior portion of the upper trapezius, roll a soft fist around the circumference of the lateral neck to draw the tissue of the superficial cylinder posteriorly.

Engage with middle knuckles (proximal interphalangeal joints) the anterior edge of the SCM, the strong yellow muscle (figure 8.38). Slowly roll your fist around the contour of the neck, maintaining your engagement with the tissue at the level of the fascia colli superficialis, and therefore also working with the anterior portion of the upper trapezius. Attention to the viscera (until the client has made at least thirty degrees of rotation), a broad area of contact with consistent pressure into the superficial tissues, and a direct run around the equator of the neck are all key to this very important move. Those with small hands working on large necks may find it advisable to do this in two strokes, one at the level of the mastoid process, and one tracking closer to the collarbone.

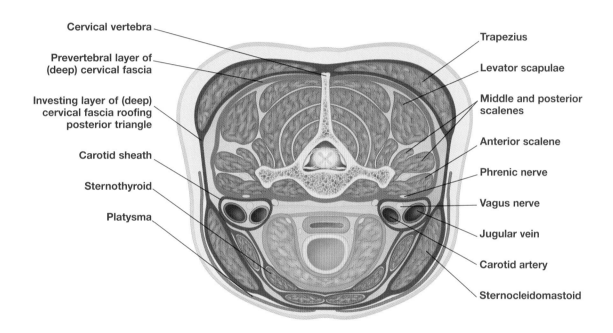

Figure 8.38: The pressure used for both techniques is just enough to engage the fascial layer of the SCM and upper trapezius and should not sink deeper into the tissue to avoid the underlying vessels. With the head rotated, as in 8.39 overleaf, the transverse processes should be underlying the line of the SCM and will therefore push the vein and artery anteriorly from the line of your pressure.

With the client's head fully turned to one side, you can then engage the SCM with a soft and relaxed fist along its full length. In this position the more delicate blood vessels will no longer be deep to the muscle, and it is safer to work with. If you are unsure of the client's history, if they are unable to turn their neck to full range, or if they have a history of dizzy spells, fainting, double vision or confusion, then it is more prudent to omit this technique until they have been checked for vertebral artery insufficiency by a proficient medical practitioner.

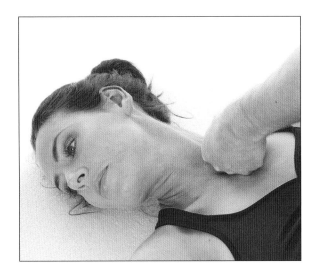 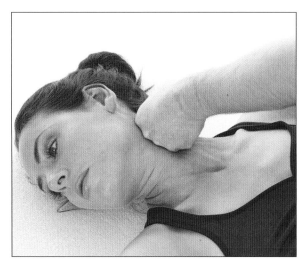

Figure 8.39a & b: Carefully engage the layer of the SCM with the proximal knuckles and guide the tissue superiorly toward the mastoid process, taking care not to either sink deeper than the muscular layer, work anteriorly to it or press into the styloid process, which lies between the mastoid process and the ear.

Engage the tissue at the inferior end with the proximal knuckles (metacarpophalangeal joints) and glide along its length toward the mastoid process. The technique can be extended over the bone if comfortable to do so, but it may be more client-friendly to swap for your fingers when working on the skull. The intention is to first lengthen and free the fascia of the SCM and then to release any adhesions of its tissue from the cranium, loosening the scalp as far as the asterion (the sutural conjunction of the parietal, occipital, and temporal bones).

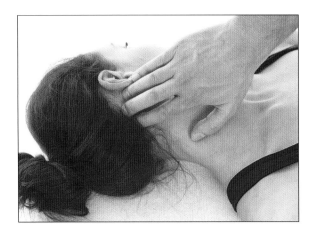

Figure 8.40: The release can be extended onto the scalp fascia to ensure all of the tissue around and above the mastoid process is also free and malleable.

Trapezius Roll (SBAL)

With your client seated, stand to one side of them, with one soft fist slightly anterior to the front edge of the trapezius and the other fist toward the posterior plane of the crest of the shoulder. Then simply roll your fists back and down, using your body as much as possible. The aim is to roll the tissue of the whole thin sheet of the trapezius (part of the superficial cylinder), but especially the anterior portion, posteriorly, helping with shoulder and neck positioning. The client can increase the stretch by leaning their head away from you or turning toward you.

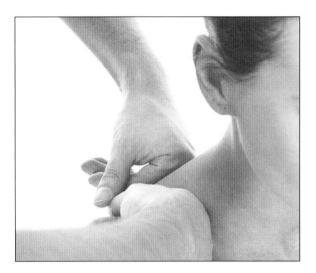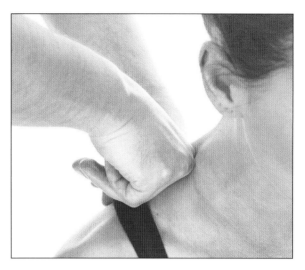

Figure 8.41a & b: The anterior fist engages the front of the upper trapezius, the posterior fist begins the stroke just behind the midline, and both guide the tissue posteriorly.

Trapezius Opening (SBAL)

With the client supine, the therapist can easily isolate a stretch into different portions of the upper trapezius. Locking into any aspect of the 'hood' of this muscle with a soft fist, the head can then be taken to the opposite side, passively or actively, to get very specific tissue stretches. To focus on the anterior portion, ipsilateral rotation can be used. Straight side flexion will be better for the crest of the muscle, and the head could be lifted slightly into flexion for the posterior element. In this position we can focus on whichever element of the upper trapezius needs greater attention.

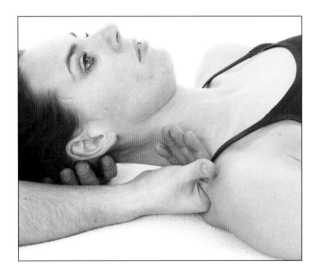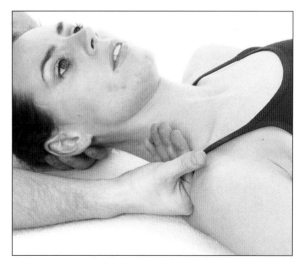

Figure 8.42a & b: Use a soft fist to lock the tissue and glide the client's head into lateral flexion. Rotation and/or flexion can be added to gain extra precision of the technique.

Opening the Suboccipital Region and Splenius Capitis and Cervicis (SBL / SPL)

Walking through life with your head a little in front of yourself puts extra strain on the tissue at the back of the head and can create much restriction in the tissue around the base of the occiput. Time can be well spent in opening this area, preparing it for the deeper work into the suboccipitals. Quite a few muscles attach along the nuchal lines – trapezius, upper erector spinae, splenius capitis – and they will all be carrying quite a bit of strain into their respective fascial connections along the base of the occiput. You can clean along these by engaging progressively deeper layers with the fingertips, and having the client turn their head to draw the tissue through your fingers against resistance.

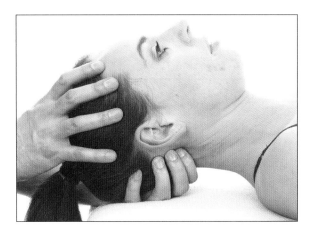 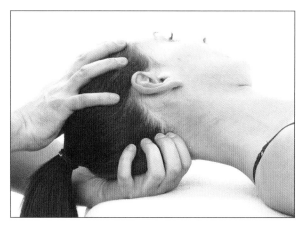

Figure 8.43a & b: Starting just behind the mastoid process, engage the tissue along the nuchal lines, and resist the movement of the tissue as your client turns their head to the opposite side. Position your fingers for minimal hair pulling, but stay up with the nuchal line for best results.

You can also release the tissue inferiorly by engaging your fingertips along the level of the nuchal lines and slowly straightening your fingers to take the tissue downward.

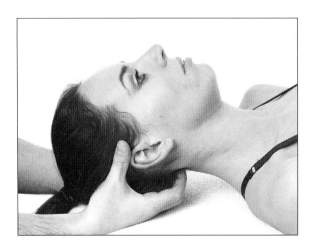 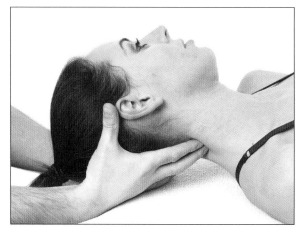

Figure 8.44a & b: With the fingers curled, the tips sink into the occipital attachments of the splenius muscles and draw them downward, as the client turns their head to the opposite side. The client can assist by gently tilting their head downward to increase the stretch in the tissue. This technique takes extension strength in your fingers which builds with practice.

The splenius muscles can be involved in tilts and rotations of the head to the same side and shifts to the opposite. For this reason you may choose to work both sides differently.

Suboccipitals (SBL)

This group of small muscles is hugely important for proprioception. They constantly monitor and assess the balance of the head on the cervical vertebrae, working to keep the eyes and ears oriented to the horizon or whatever else engages your attention, and contracting in anticipation of any change in the center of gravity.

When we look at the subocciptals from the side (figure 8.12c), we can get a better view of their separate functions. The rectus capitis posterior major travels slightly laterally from the spinous process of C2. It is, however, quite vertical compared to the smaller rectus capitis posterior minor, which travels from the deeper C1 back to the occipital attachment. It is at a similar angle to the obliquus capitis superior, which travels back from the transverse processes of the atlas to the lateral aspect of the nuchal lines. Both of these muscles will be shortened in anterior head positions. Rectus capitis posterior major and obliquus capitis inferior will be involved with rotations of the head and C1/C2. Rectus capitis posterior major will also be shortened in cases of a posterior tilt of the head, such as often occurs with spectacle wearers, particularly people who wear bifocals.

To locate each of the superior suboccipitals, sink the tips of your index, middle and ring fingers deep to the occiput, each ring finger either side of the ligamentum nuchae and inferior to the external occipital protuberance. Allow your fingers to travel deep and then curl them back toward you, superiorly onto the inferior surface of the occiput. If you strum back and forth, you should hopefully feel the 'speed bump' (occasionally short string) of the larger and more superficial rectus capitis posterior major under your middle finger. You can help this muscle lengthen by hooking the tip of your middle finger into the belly of the muscle, locking in an inferior direction, and then asking your client to gently nod their head (anteriorly tilting it), to create a stretch.

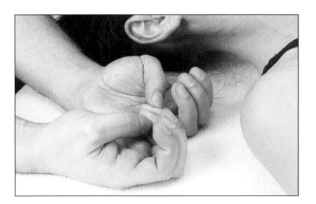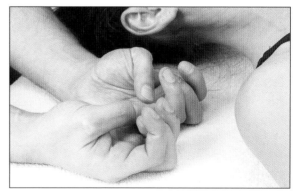

Figure 8.45a & b: Here we see the finger placement to find the upper three suboccipitals. The middle finger then drops away to focus the work on the rectus capitis posterior minor and the obliquus capitis superior.

By dropping your middle finger away from the tissue and allowing your index and ring fingers to sink deeper and fold back, you should be contacting the rectus capitis posterior minor under your ring finger and the obliquus capitis superior under your index finger. To work with these muscles and to create a deep relaxation in the system, drop your hands into the foam of the massage table to glide the occiput posteriorly on the atlas. Then (and only then) slowly bring the occiput superiorly to open the shortened fascia.

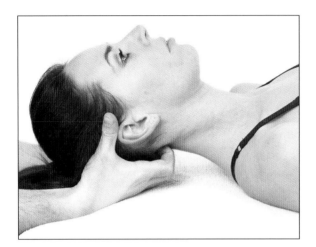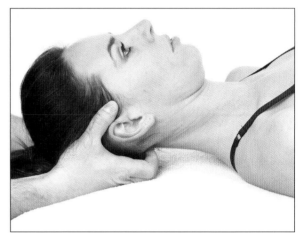

Figure 8.46a & b: With your fingertips placed on the inferior aspect of the occiput, draw the head down into the table and then slowly superiorly toward the top of the table.

This technique can be done in phases. Take up the slack by performing the two previous movements, which should be combined to create a fluid 'scoop'. Then wait for the relaxation, take up the further slack, and again wait for the tissue to ease before increasing the movement slightly.

Scalenes

This group of important muscles helps stabilize the neck from different angles, but will therefore also help create a range of patterns in terms of structural balance. The anterior scalenes will pull the neck forward and down, maybe with a rotation if one side overcomes the other. The middle and posterior scalenes will draw the neck to one side, creating a lateral shift or tilt.

The anterior scalenes are tucked deep to, and partly obscured by, the sternocleidomastoid. Access them by sliding your fingers under the SCM, roughly halfway along the neck. The nail side of your fingertips should be against the deep aspect of the SCM and the pads will rest on the upper portion of the anterior scalenes. You can now glide down the line of the muscle toward the first rib, as the client pushes into their feet (knees up) and lets their head slide along the couch toward you, flattening the cervical lordosis to elongate the target muscles.

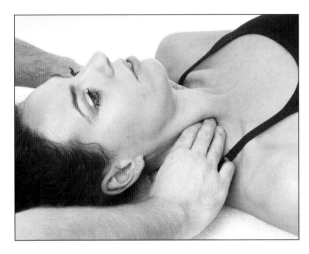
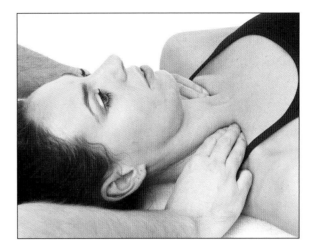

Figure 8.47a & b: Gently ease your fingers deep to the SCM from the outside, asking your client to alert you if they feel any form of nerve sensation. Check your positioning as the client takes a deep breath by feeling for the contraction of the anterior scalenes below your fingertips during the inhalation. Lock into the tissue and resist as the client pushes into their feet to lengthen the back of their neck, the back of their head gliding along the table toward you and their chin drawing toward the front of the throat.

A stronger technique can be achieved by pinning the distal attachment of the muscle and, passively or actively, having the client's head turn to the same side and laterally flex to the opposite side.

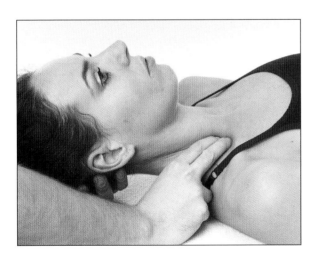
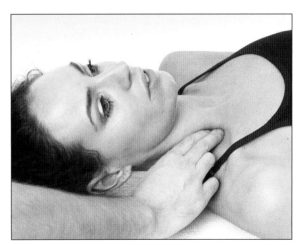

Figure 8.48a & b: Working one anterior scalene at a time, lock into the distal attachment and slowly rotate the head to the same side and laterally flex it to the opposite side.

To check that you are palpating and working on the scalenes, the tissue under your contact should feel ropey, almost like bass guitar strings. You can check by asking your client to take a deep breath. The scalenes should contract in the last five to ten percent of the inhalation, as they raise their ribs for the last little extra (though if you feel nothing happen, make sure they are actually going the whole way; if they have respiratory issues, they may be contracting earlier or already be under strain).

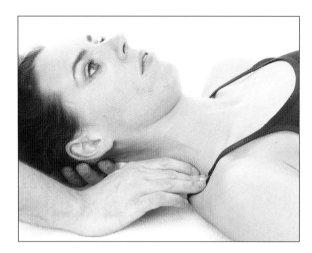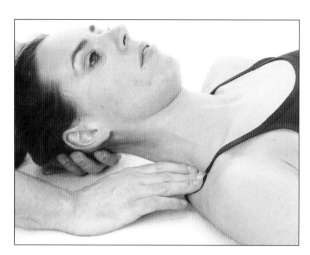

Figure 8.49a & b: The middle and posterior scalenes can be found deep to the trapezius. Fold your fingers under the front edge of the muscle and you should feel the strings of the muscles coming down from the transverse processes to the ribs.

With your fingers folded deep to the anterior portion of the upper trapezius, you can pin the distal attachments of the middle and posterior scalenes using the tips of one or two fingers, as you instruct the client to glide their head to the opposite side. To target the posterior scalene, a little head and neck rotation to the opposite side may help increase the stretch slightly.

Please note: The scalenes are intimate with the brachial plexus, which exits the neck via the gap between the anterior and middle scalenes. Before working this area, advise your client to inform you if they feel any form of nerve sensation. Should this happen, you know your pressure is between the anterior and middle scalene, so simply change the position or angle of your contact and recheck. In those where the fascia is especially bound, some brachial plexus involvement in the initial stages of freeing the scalenes is inevitable. By moderating your pressure in tune with their sensation, the fascia binding the plexus to the myofascia can be freed and the nerve sensation will progressively disappear.

The Shoulder and Arm

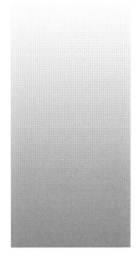

9

The Shoulder

The human shoulder and arm are unique in the animal world. We have heard a lot about the opposable thumb and how that made *Homo habilis*, the 'handy man'. Our singular abilities and biopsychology, however, rest on the manner in which the whole shoulder and arm connect into the rest of us, not just our thumb. Similar eye-hand coordination may show up in other primates – like the chimpanzees who use reeds to extract termites – but in humans the manipulation of the world has extended into language.

The structure of our language – subject/verb/object – is surely based around the fact that we have hands that change and move those objects in the world. It would be easy to imagine that equally large-brained dolphins and whales – with flippers instead of hands, and eyes on the side of the head – would construct a very different syntax.

A Brief History of the Shoulder

The shoulders have managed a wide variety of structural arrangements in their history. The shoulder assembly probably started as a pectoral fin sticking sideways out of a fish. Its job then was to stabilize and act as a rudder for the fish in the water, while the spine provided the main propulsion. As the fish crawled out on land (or, to be more accurate, as the waters receded and some fish were forced out), those with fins that were located more toward the front of the creature succeeded better, as this position allowed the fins to touch the mud and be active in propulsion and steering, thus preserving stability in the 'air' world.

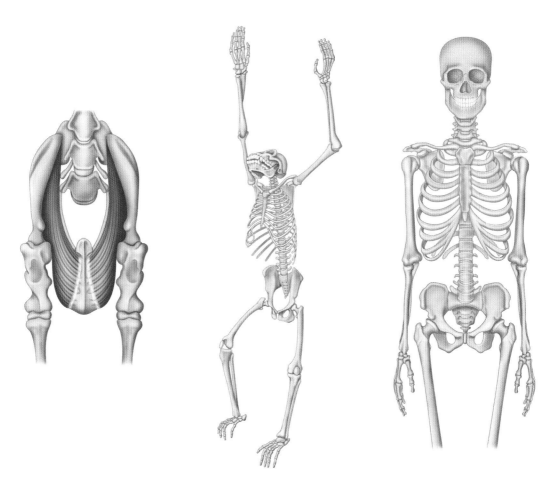

Figure 9.1: The shoulder has a varied history – from a fin, to supporting most of our bodyweight in compression, to supporting our weight in tension, and finally to its own weight being supported on the trunk.

Being very unexacting zoologically, we can see a general line of development from these humble beginnings. In the amphibian, the whole arm tends to be flat on the floor, as if you were to lie on your belly with your arm out to your side, palm down. This extends the 'fin' into that world and allows the action of the spine to be extended into the environment for increased traction and leverage.

In the alligator and his ilk, the arm has bent at the elbow, so that the upper arm comes straight out, and the lower arm straight down so that the 'palm' rests on the ground beside the trunk. This is more precise in motivation than the amphibian leg; but because it is out to the side, it still cannot lift the alligator torso off the ground for long.

The predominant mammalian pattern sees the shoulders protracting and flexing horizontally to bring the straight arm in under the body, making it easier to lift the torso off the ground. This 'popular' arrangement – employed by horses, cats, dogs, lions, etc. – uses the shoulder as the primary weight-bearing limb. In these animals, the foreleg is therefore usually fairly straight compared to the hind leg, which is often bent at more angles to give it a better mechanical advantage for powerful pushing and jumping. The shoulder sits atop a foreleg that is straight and therefore able to resist the weight of the large upper body.

For this pattern to work, the rib cage actually lies in a sling, made predominantly from the serratus anterior and attendant fascia, which runs from the medial border of the scapula under the ribs. This arrangement does not require a collarbone; in fact it actively discourages having one, as a cat wants the shoulder-blade as close to the center of the body as possible. Right up through the gorilla, the rib cage of most quadrupeds is comparatively narrow from right to left, and deep from front to back.

The arboreal monkey, presumably in our family 'tree', used the same bones and muscles, but added in the collarbone, to create an entirely different manner of support – namely supporting the bodyweight in tension by hanging it off a branch from the arm. In this 'new' arrangement, the range of usable movement is facilitated by moving the shoulder away from the center line with a wider rib cage and the scapula pushed yet wider by the clavicle. The fascia of the arm connects up in a different way to transfer the tension from section to section without so much tensile strain on the joint ligaments.

In the horse shoulder, the weight conveys primarily through the bones, with the soft tissues as stabilizers (more like our leg). In the brachiating ape, the tension transfers primarily through the soft tissue sinew (explaining how the soft tissue connections which we are about to explore in our arms – even with very similar arrangement of bones and muscles – are connected up so very differently from our legs).

Our own human shoulders are yet another mechanism employing the same bones and muscles. They sit like a yoke on the rib cage, as well as hang from the head and spine, asking for postural support rather than giving it. When called upon to work or play, they do so nimbly in either tension or compression in a wide variety of positions: gripping a hammer or a racquet, clasping a violin or an épée, clipping on a necklace or squat-pressing a barbell, flaring in a swan dive or poising over a computer keyboard.

Compressive Forces in the Shoulder

Though the human shoulder is designed to work in this way, the complexity of the limb and its high mobility that allows the girdle to be placed in so many different ways also makes for easy postural malpositioning – the primary underlying cause of shoulder or neck injury. So this chapter will focus on the proper positioning of the scapula, which is the key to many of the dysfunctions that plague our 'well-armed' society.

The scapula is just one of a dozen or so choice points (joints) between the fingertips and the ribs and spine of the axial skeleton. Lots of mobility creates lots of opportunity for misuse. So before we look at the scapular muscles in detail, let us follow the flow of compressive force out of the arm to see that biomechanically the arm is much longer than it looks.

Whereas there is no formal 'joint' between a horse's arm (foreleg) bones and the rest of his skeleton, in our arm the addition of a clavicle does create an axial-appendicular connection at the sternoclavicular joint at the top of the manubrium of the sternum. Put your fingertips at the top of the sternum and take your shoulder girdle in a circle to feel this shallow saddle joint circumduct.

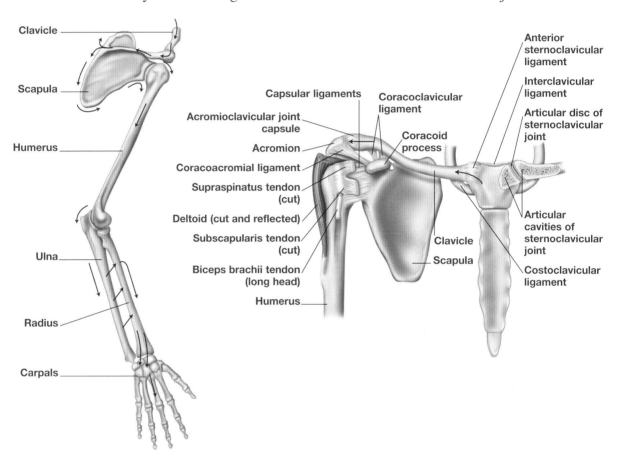

Figure 9.2: Force tracks its way up or down the shoulder and arm in a convoluted way, which we need to understand in treating the sequelae to compressive injuries to the arm.

From here, we follow the collarbone out to the acromioclavicular joint (which can be felt as a little valley about three centimeters (one inch) in from the tip of the shoulder), which transfers the force into the acromion of the scapula. But if we follow the bone from here, our fingers (and the force) go back along the scapular spine to the medial border, where we go both superiorly and inferiorly along that edge to gather in the blade of the bone and the accompanying rotator cuff muscles to traverse the glenohumeral joint into the humerus.

The humerus is a straight shot to the elbow, but then it starts to get complicated again. The humerus transfers directly into the ulna, but the ulna has very little contact with the carpal bones in the wrist (known formally as the radiocarpal joint). Instead, the force transmits from the ulna via the interosseous membrane to the radius, and from the radius to the first row of three carpals, and then to the second four, and on out to the hand. (Compare this to the leg, where the weight transfer is direct from the femur to the tibia to the talus, leaving the fibula as an extra, non-weight-bearing strut.) The interosseous membrane thus acts as a shock absorber for the impact of catching a ball, or landing on your hand in a fall.

Thus the forces that run through the arm – out from our muscular thrust, or in from impact – take a circuitous route that absorbs shock and distributes strain around the system. Malpositioning of the shoulder disturbs this delicate system, which then directs the shock into tissues that are not prepared to handle it, and thus makes injuries more likely. The mobility of the scapula, and its crucial role in transferring force in a circuitous route from the humerus to the clavicle or vice-versa, makes it a frequent key to re-establishing shoulder integrity.

The Muscles of the Shoulder Girdle

Obviously the fascial length and neuromuscular tension in the muscles that hold all these bones is going to determine the positioning of the bones, so it is to these muscles that we turn our attention. We will spend more time with the core muscles of the shoulder – those that set underlying position – and less with the more well-known, superficial, coordinating muscles of the trapezius, latissimus dorsi, pectorals, and deltoids.

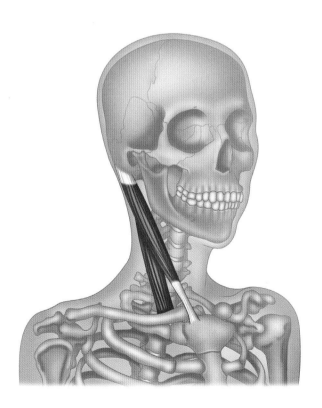

The clavicle, that Johnny-come-lately strut unique to apes and us, has only three muscles that connect it to the axial skeleton: the subclavius, the occipito-clavicular portion of the trapezius, and the clavicular head of the sternocleidomastoid (SCM). Taking the last first, the clavicular head of the SCM has very little effect on the position of the clavicle, either in posture or in action, because it attaches so close to the axis of the sternoclavicular joint. It is primarily a mover of the neck and head, and its clavicular attachment is practically as immovable as its sternal attachment. Therefore the SCM can be safely ignored as a shoulder muscle.

Figure 9.3: The sternocleidomastoideus muscle has little effect on the shoulder due to its attachment close to the sternoclavicular joint.

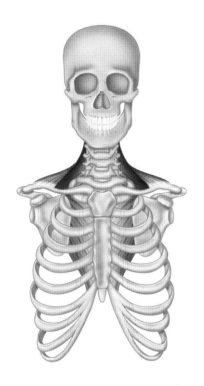

The anterior edge of the trapezius, however, is another story. Attached to the distal end of the clavicle, the trapezius is of course a major mover of the shoulder girdle. This anterior edge of the trapezius lifts the outer end of the collarbone up, as in a shrug. Constant tension in this muscle will either give the clavicles a characteristic 'V' shape (instead of the 'proper' straight line) when viewed from the front or it may end up pulling the head forward.

Figure 9.4: The trapezius, on the other hand, strongly lifts the outer tip of the collarbone with its leading edge.

The subclavius is often listed as a depressor of the clavicle, but how often does your clavicle get depressed? One look at the subclavius shows us that the muscle is nearly parallel to the long axis of the bone. This suggests that the primary purpose of the subclavius is to reinforce the joint – a muscular ligament, if you will, that tethers the clavicle into its shallow joint with the sternum.

The subclavius should allow a little glide in the sternoclavicular joint. If it is too muscularly or (more frequently) fascially tightened, you will see the shoulder-blades lift when the arms are spread wide. If the subclavius is too muscularly or fascially loose (rare, and often the result of an injury), the clavicle will not be stable, and other muscles around the scapula will be tense to compensate.

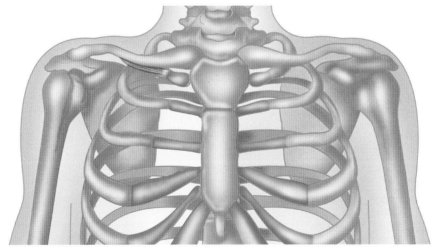

Figure 9.5: The subclavius muscle is a tether for the collarbone.

If we turn our attention now to the mobile scapula resting on the posterior rib cage, we find many more muscles coming in from every direction, suspending the scapula within many tensional spokes: levator scapulae, rhomboid minor, rhomboid major, the nine slips of serratus anterior, tiny omohyoid, pectoralis minor, sometimes latissimus dorsi, and the overlying trapezius pulling from three different directions at once. The scapula is passively held and moved within the balance of these many muscles; but how do we make sense of all these competing pulls?

The Scapular 'X'

In considering all the muscles that hold the scapula to the axial skeleton (we will consider the muscles that hold the scapula to the humerus – like the rotator cuff – later in this chapter), we can see an 'X' of muscles that are primarily responsible for scapular position. Learn to see and treat the myofascia of this 'X' and you will have little trouble with getting the scapula to rest in its biomechanically sound position.

Although people vary, the best resting position for the scapula is achieved when the medial border is parallel to the spinous processes, about on the angle of the ribs and vertical when viewed from the side (i.e. like a cliff, not a roof).

One leg of this powerful 'X' is formed by the rhomboids and the serratus anterior muscle. The rhomboids (we take major and minor together here) tether the medial border of the scapula to the spinous processes of the upper thoracic vertebrae and lower cervical vertebrae, pulling the medial border up and in. The serratus anterior pulls the medial border down and out toward the lateral ribs. In fact, you could say that there is really one large strap of muscle – the 'rhombo-serratus' muscle – in which the medial border of the scapula floats.

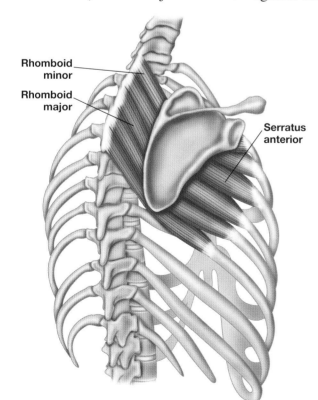

Rhomboid minor

Rhomboid major

Serratus anterior

Figure 9.6: The two rhomboids and the serratus anterior in reality form one myofascial sling that holds the scapula in place.

If the serratus anterior is concentrically loaded or locked into a shortened position, then the shoulder-blade will be low and lateral on the rib cage – think of a weight-lifter or someone with a kyphotic spine. In this case, the rhomboids will be overstretched, eccentrically loaded, or locked into a lengthened position. Those rhomboids will be full of trigger points and complaints, but it is the serratus anterior that needs lengthening work. If the rhomboids are concentrically loaded, the serratus anterior will be overstretched, and the shoulder-blades will be more medial than the angle of the ribs. This pattern often, but not always, accompanies a decreased thoracic curve or *flatback*.

Occasionally one sees the pattern of both parts of the rhombo-serratus being locked short, usually as part of a short Spiral Line, of which the rhombo-serratus is a part. In these cases, the scapula rides high on the back, and the whole shoulder girdle appears small for the body. These clients need loosening work on both sides of the rhomboid-serratus equation.

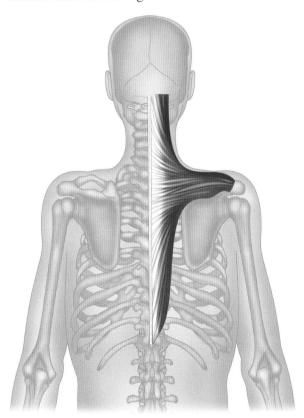

If this leg of the scapular 'X' involves the up-and-in or down-and-out option, then the other leg must involve the down-and-in or up-and-out option. The down-and-in part is easy to see; the lower triangle of the trapezius from about T5 to T12 pulls down and in where the scapular spine meets the medial border. The latissimus dorsi sometimes has a fascial connection to the inferior angle of the scapula, which can in these cases help to keep the scapula down and in as well.

Figure 9.7: The lower trapezius pulls down and in from the medial border of the scapula. Sometimes the latissimus dorsi can help with this motion too, if it is connected to the scapula.

Surely, however, no muscle can pull up and out from the acromion? None does, but if we go over the shoulder like a backpack strap, we find the small but powerful pectoralis minor pulling down and in on the front, and this has the same effect on the scapula, lifting it on the ribs, pulling it laterally, bringing it around the ribs, and tilting it anteriorly.

These are all elements of the common term *protraction*, but we do well to separate these elements to specify the treatment options for the pectoralis minor specifically and the scapular complex in general.

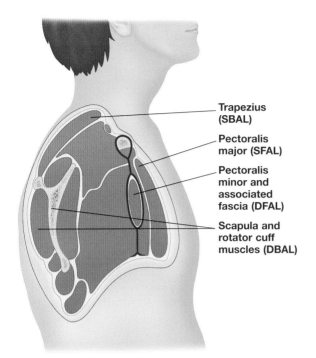

Trapezius
(SBAL)

Pectoralis
major (SFAL)

Pectoralis
minor and
associated
fascia (DFAL)

Scapula and
rotator cuff
muscles (DBAL)

The pectoralis minor tethers the scapula from the front, attaching from the upper ribs (listed as three to five in many books, but in practice often ribs 2 to 5) to the coracoid process. The coracoid process is a little thumb of bone that sticks through to the front from the blade of the scapula to provide an attachment point for flexors of the arm and the pectoralis minor. When in good working order, the pectoralis minor provides a mobile restraining pivot for the scapular movement created by the larger superficial muscles.

Figure 9.8: The pectoralis minor tethers the scapula onto the front of the rib cage.

All too often, however, this muscle is not in good working order, and is either fascially short (it lives in the clavipectoral fascia, a sheet almost as big as the overlying pectoralis major) or muscularly contracted. Either type of shortness can affect the ability of the shoulder to flex fully (as in older people who have trouble reaching the top shelf) and can affect breathing negatively, as well as pulling the scapula out of position up and over the rib cage.

From a muscle training point of view, the solution to the imbalance in this leg of the 'X' would be to tone the lower trapezius, with the various kinds of rowing exercises. This is a good idea for almost everyone who drives or sits at a computer for any significant amount of time, but we urge you to first consider stretching and opening of the pectoralis minor area before training the trapezius; this will make the exercise more successful in changing posture, and easier to maintain. In the Western industrialized population with which we are accustomed to working, the opposite pattern – where the lower trapezius is too short and the pectoralis minor is overly stretched – is rare indeed.

Aside from these four, there are other muscular *spokes* around the scapular hub. The omohyoid is difficult to palpate, and too small to have much effect on either the function or the position of the shoulder. The levator scapulae, however, is a frequent contributor to scapular stress.

Our clients come in complaining of stress and point to their upper shoulders. The attachment point of the levator scapulae at the superior angle of the scapula is almost universally sore to the inquiring fingers. Why stress goes here is a worthwhile question to ask. For the answer, we must turn the body to the side and look at the head position.

If the neck is straight and the head is balanced over the rib cage, the head can be supported and rotated by a complex of two axial muscles: the splenius muscles and the SCMs, assisted and guided by the deeper and smaller muscles of the motor cylinder, by the suboccipital complex at the very middle.

If – for reasons of anxiety, literal short sightedness, or injury – the head starts to go forward, this complex of axial muscles is unbalanced, and they lose their ability to keep the head poised and mobile atop the neck. In these cases, shoulder muscles are recruited to stabilize the head and neck, which leads to strain problems for both the neck and the shoulder. Correcting this problem frees both the neck and shoulder from parasitic tension that sets the long-term stage for degenerative disease in the neck and injury in the shoulder.

Looking at the neck from the side, we can see the 'proper' balance of forces between the two sets of SCMs and splenius capitis and cervicis muscles. But we can also see a similar 'X' formed from shoulder muscles: the leading edge of the trapezius can recapitulate the SCM, and the poor levator scapulae, in head-forward posture, becomes the 'capitis-preventus-going-forwardus', constantly strained because it becomes a tether for the heavy head, not simply a lifter of the shoulder-blade as its name implies.

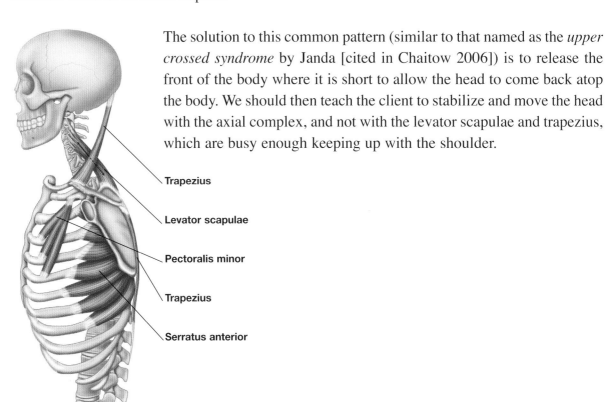

The solution to this common pattern (similar to that named as the *upper crossed syndrome* by Janda [cited in Chaitow 2006]) is to release the front of the body where it is short to allow the head to come back atop the body. We should then teach the client to stabilize and move the head with the axial complex, and not with the levator scapulae and trapezius, which are busy enough keeping up with the shoulder.

Trapezius

Levator scapulae

Pectoralis minor

Trapezius

Serratus anterior

Figure 9.9: The head 'should' be supported by the axial splenius capitis and the SCM, but often shoulder muscles – frequently the pictured upper trapezius and levator scapulae muscles – are recruited as substitutes.

From the shoulder on out to the fingertips, we will organize our journey through the anatomy in terms of the myofascial meridians of the arm.

The Arm Lines

Although the arms and the legs clearly echo each other, the anatomy of the arms is more complex than that of the legs, due to the arm's extra mobility. In order to make this complexity manageable, we will describe the arm's anatomy in terms of four myofascial continuities, a bit like kinetic chains, that traverse the arm from the spine and ribs all the way out to the fingers. There are many details of arm anatomy that we cannot include as they would swamp this book were we to cover them all. But we can use these lines to see the overall layout of the arm, to which you can add more details as you find the need to put them in.

All four Arm Lines – Superficial Front, Deep Front, Deep Back and Superficial Back – run the full length of the arm from the axial center to the tips of the fingers. They are named for how they are in relation to the armpit: The Superficial Front Arm Line (SFAL) includes the pectoralis major on the front of the chest. The Deep Front Arm Line (DFAL) includes the pectoralis minor and subclavius in the clavipectoral fascia in the front of the armpit deep to the pectoralis major. The Deep Back Arm Line (DBAL) includes the whole rotator cuff in the back of the armpit. The Superficial Back Arm Line (SBAL) includes the trapezius lying over the rotator cuff in the very back of the armpit.

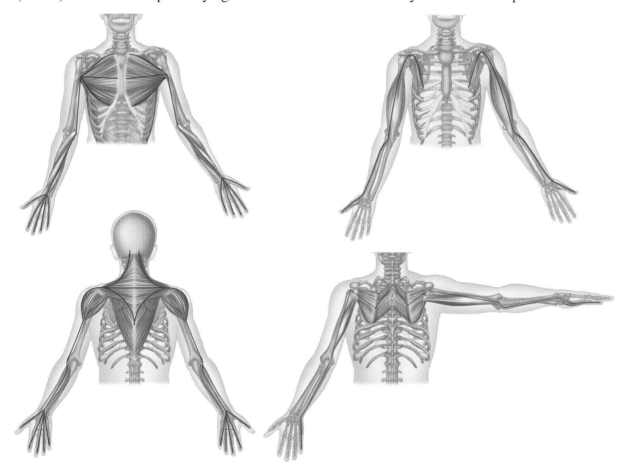

Figure 9.10: The four Arm Lines are arranged in order as they pass on either side of the axilla on their way to the four 'corners' of the hand.

Let us begin with the SFAL. Hold your arm out to the side, elbow down, palm facing front. The SFAL now lies along the front of your arm. Follow along in your own body as we trace it. The SFAL starts (or ends, your call) on the pads of your five fingers, drawing through the palm of your hand with all the superficial and deep finger flexors which pass through the carpal tunnel and down into the underside of your arm. (Interestingly, the longest-reaching muscles here are the deepest, whereas in other parts of the body the longer muscles tend to be on the surface, with the shorter ones underlying.)

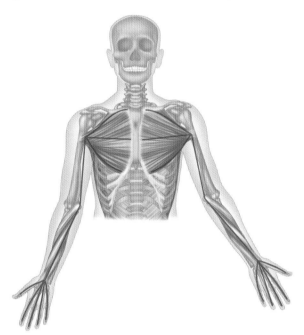

Figure 9.11: The Superficial Front Arm Line.

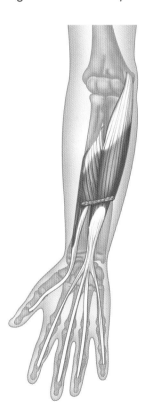

From here we include the flexors of the wrist, the flexor carpi ulnaris and radialis, which join in with these finger flexors to bind together at the common flexor tendon, easily found at the medial humeral epicondyle on the inside of your elbow. Strum just proximally to this bony landmark to feel a cord going up the upper arm. This cord is part of the medial intermuscular septum, a fascial strip that separates the biceps brachii and flexors from the triceps brachii. This provides the fascial connection from the hand and finger flexors to the distal attachment of the pectoralis major and the latissimus dorsi.

Figure 9.12: The many forearm flexors – like the flexor digitorum superficialis – bind together at the medial humeral epicondyle.

You may well ask what the 'widest muscle of the back' is doing in the Front Arm lines, but the latissimus dorsi attaches to the front of the humerus and is thus connected to this line. It turns out that latissimus dorsi starts its embryological life more on the front of the body (ventral) and migrates posteriorly during development, so there is some method in this madness. Practically, the two muscles together – latissimus dorsi and pectoralis major – give the SFAL a very wide origin on the rib cage, the back and even the hip. This gives us a very broad set of controls over the arm, especially in throwing and catching.

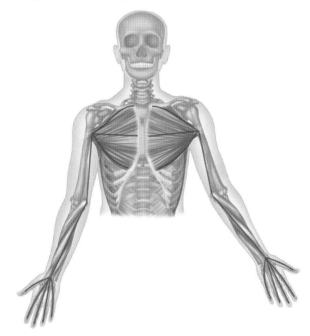

Figure 9.13: The SFAL has a very wide origin on the rib cage for maximum control over the throwing and manipulating arm.

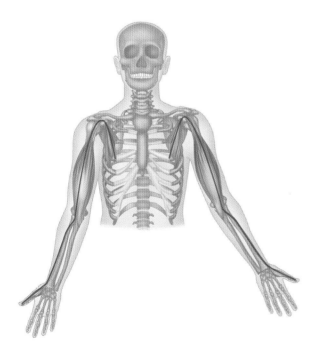

We move now to the DFAL. This is most easily visualized by holding your arm out with the elbow pointed back and the palm facing the ground. Reach around with your other hand and grab your thumb. This line passes from the thumb through those thenar muscles at the base of the thumb, along the fascia on the outside of the radius. It disappears in the 'meat' of the flexors and extensors, only to re-emerge at the inside of the elbow with the biceps brachii.

Figure 9.14: The Deep Front Arm Line.

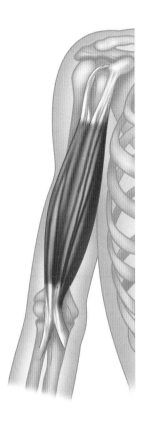

Find the tendon of your biceps brachii at the crook of your elbow, and notice that it buries itself into your arm to meet the radius. Two muscles on either side of the tendon make a 'V' around it: the pronator teres and the supinator. These two muscles, which essentially control the angle of the thumb via the radius, are included in this line.

The biceps brachii goes up the inner surface of the arm and splits into two heads. The long head goes around the head of the humerus and inserts into the top of the shoulder joint; more on this later. The short head runs up and into the coracoid process of the scapula. Two muscles underlie the biceps brachii. The brachialis crosses only the elbow, and can be felt bulging under the biceps brachii on either side of its tendon when flexing the elbow against resistance. The coracobrachialis crosses on the shoulder and acts principally to adduct the elbow against the body. Those whose elbow rests closer to the torso than the wrist need work in this muscle.

Figure 9.15: The biceps brachii, with its two heads and two 'feet', is really a crossover muscle among three of the Arm Lines, but it is principally part of the DFAL.

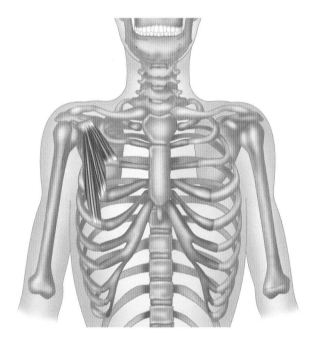

The last link in the chain of the DFAL is the pectoralis minor, which runs from the coracoid process (and is strongly fascially linked across this attachment with both the biceps and the coracobrachialis) to the third through fifth ribs in the front. Looking fascially, we can see that the pectoralis minor is sandwiched in the much larger clavipectoral fascia that also surrounds the subclavius. We have already covered these important muscles above.

Figure 9.16: The pectoralis minor, the link from the appendicular part of the DFAL to the axial, plays a key role in this line, and in shoulder function in general.

The DFAL controls the thumb, which controls the grip. It also stabilizes the arm so that the SFAL can impart momentum to a ball (or to us, if we are up on the parallel bars or leaping a wall). It is important for bodyworkers doing thumb work (say, in trigger point release) to keep this line open and connected, lest we put too much pressure into the base of the thumb.

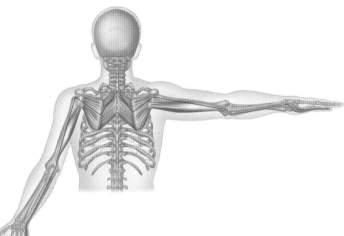

If the DFAL is the leading edge of the arm's 'wing', controlling the grip and meeting the buffeting winds, then the DBAL is its complement, controlling the trailing edge and stabilizing the outside of the arm. The DBAL is most easily visualized by putting your arm out to the side with the elbow pointing back and the palm down; the DBAL is now arranged along the posterior side of your arm.

Figure 9.17: The Deep Back Arm Line.

Beginning distally, the fascia alongside the little finger leads to the hypothenar muscles along the outside of the heel of the hand. The line continues up the fascia of the ulna to the olecranon, where it joins the triceps brachii. This muscle group carries us up the back of the arm to the outer end of the scapula. Here we pick up the entire 'scapula sandwich' of the rotator cuff, which we discuss further in a moment. The final links in this chain are the levator scapulae and the rhomboids, about which we have already spoken.

The structure and function of the rotator cuff requires a bit of attention here. The blade of the scapula is very thin; it simply provides a large attachment area for the large and strong muscles that at once reinforce the capsule of the shoulder and 'point' the arm, the way the body controls the eye.

The shoulder is the most moveable joint in the body. If you cut the capsule to break the vacuum seal, you could pull the humerus almost two centimeters (two-thirds of one inch) from the glenoid cavity of the scapula. This mobility requires corresponding stability, so the tendons of the supraspinatus, infraspinatus, teres minor and subscapularis blend into the capsular ligaments, providing adjustable support that can loosen to allow full movement of the shoulder, or tighten to reinforce the joint's stability. The capsule itself is weak in the anterior portion (which is why your older brother twisting your arm behind your back is so persuasive), and the joint is not reinforced by a muscle below (which is why you wear shoulder pads in American football).

The four cuff muscles cover the back, top and sides of the humeral head. The teres minor and infraspinatus cover the back side, and assist the posterior deltoid in laterally rotating the humerus, or resisting medial rotation (quite a job, considering the number and strength of the shoulder's medial rotators). It is hard to miss infraspinatus, with its slick fascial covering and sufficient bulk to cover the whole lower part of the scapula, but the tiny teres minor is worth finding, as this small muscle tethers the humerus posteriorly. Feel under the infraspinatus tendon, about halfway between the posterior edge of the acromion and the fold of the armpit skin in the back. Strum to find a strong little muscle, usually about the size of the client's little finger or a large pencil.

The supraspinatus is listed as a lateral rotator also; but it mostly helps out in abduction, by holding the head of the humerus down into the socket so that the deltoid (and later trapezius) can abduct smoothly. Thus, it lies on top of the joint, filling in that fossa above the spine. The fossa is roughly two centimeters (two-thirds of one inch) deep; so if you want to wake up or really lengthen the supraspinatus, it is necessary to get down into this fossa to affect this muscle. A couple of passes over its surface often does not get the job done.

The subscapularis lines the entire front of the scapula, and is the only medial rotator of the group. This is a multipennate muscle with several tendons, so do not expect to get it smoothed out entirely. But it is often muscularly tight, and even more often fascially tied to the underlying serratus anterior, so it is definitely worth the time to free it for full functioning.

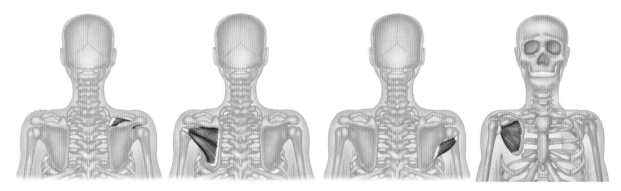

Figure 9.18: The four muscles of the rotator cuff 'point' the arm, in the same way the body points the eye at the object of its attention; from left to right, supraspinatus, infraspinatus, teres minor, and subscapularis.

The four muscles taken together control the ball of the humerus, the way the four muscles around the eye 'point' the eye toward the object of your attention. This essential role requires both strength and freedom. Time spent with the rotator cuff is well rewarded in both curative and preventive results.

Our final line in the arm, the SBAL, can be visualized by putting your arm out to the side with the elbow down and the palm forward. The line runs from the fingernails up the back of the hand with all the extensors, running under the extensor retinaculum, picking up the extensor carpi ulnaris and radialis muscles to join the common extensor tendon at the lateral humeral epicondyle. The tendon can be easily felt on the back of the forearm, near the elbow.

The lateral intermuscular septum, which again divides flexors from extensors on the outside, is not so easily felt as its medial complement, but it is nevertheless dissectible from the epicondyle to the end of the deltoid. The deltoid runs from a point at the deltoid tubercle to the lateral rim of the clavicle, acromion and scapular spine. The trapezius completes the line by continuing the deltoid to the entire thoracic and cervical spine from the occiput to T12. This line provides the movement complement to the SFAL, active in backhand tennis shots and any lifting movements. It is the top of our 'wing'.

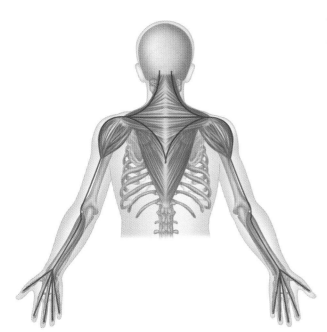

While we hope the lines help you visualize the arm anatomy in an organized way, if they seem incomplete, that is because they are. Because of the arm's variable stability and mobility requirements, some muscles, parts of muscles, or fascial structures must cross over from one line to another. To end this chapter, we list a few of the 'crossover' structures.

Figure 9.19: The Superficial Back Arm Line.

The biceps brachii is perhaps the best example: it not only has two heads but also two 'feet', so it provides two crossovers in one muscle. The short head we included in the DFAL, but the long head goes up over the humeral head to connect near the supraspinatus, thus connecting the DFAL to the DBAL. At its 'foot' end, the biceps brachii has the bicipital aponeurosis, which splays off into the flexor group. It thus connects the DFAL to the SFAL (and is therefore handy for carrying heavy objects, e.g. suitcases).

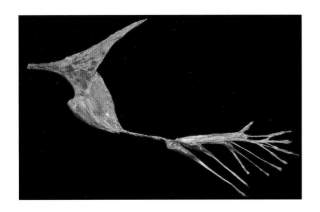

Figure 9.20: This dissection of the SBAL shows clearly how the fascia is continuous from muscle to muscle. Most anatomists aim the scalpel down and distinguish between the muscles. We turned the scalpel sideways to see how they were joined.

The brachioradialis muscle crosses between the SBAL and the DFAL, and the pronator quadratus joins the two Deep Arm Lines at the wrist. These and other structures allow the smooth functioning of the many joints of the arm in the many positions required to fix the sink, roughhouse with your child or sail a boat. The arms are a marvelous invention. Freed from supporting the body's weight, they can reach out and hug, write or heal, in the uniquely human way the brain has learnt to use the hands.

BodyReading the Shoulders

The shoulder girdles can be difficult to assess because of their many planes of movement. If we break those down individually, you will begin to get an idea of how they combine to form the myriad of patterns you can see in the street.

First of all, they can shift up or down. You can usually read this by looking at the line of the clavicles, which are normally parallel to the floor. Remember that we have to read the body parts in relation to each other, so a better way of reading this consistently would be to compare the clavicles to the line of the sternum, as they have more connections to the rib cage than they do to the floor. If the rib cage tilts, so too should the shoulder girdles, to maintain the ninety-degree angle between the clavicle and the sternum.

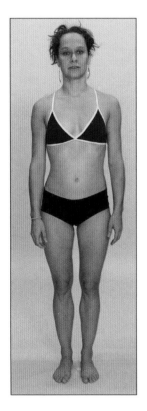
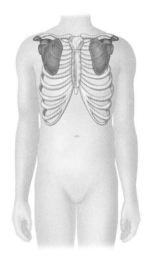
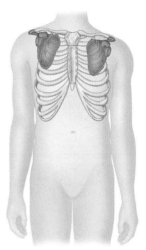
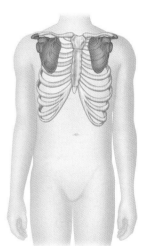

Figure 9.21a & b: For example, in (a) we can see that the right shoulder girdle is inferiorly shifted and the left shifted superiorly relative to the floor; but when we look at her rib cage, we see that it has tilted to the right. So the primary problem is with the rib cage and the soft tissue that connects it to the pelvis, rather than the soft tissue of the shoulders. In (b) we see shoulders in balance with the ribs, tilted to the left relative to the ribs and finally shoulders that look level relative to the ground but are actually right tilted relative to the thorax.

For a true superior shift we would obviously be drawn to the shoulder elevators, upper trapezius and levator scapulae. But we can also address the balance in the *rhombo-serratus* sling, one leg of the 'X' explained above. The rhomboids will help lift the girdle and the serratus anterior draw it down. This pattern is easily seen when we look at it from the back.

For an inferior shift we would need to work with the subclavius and the many depressors of the shoulder. But often we need also to ensure that the girdle is receiving support from the ribs beneath, as a common reason for a shoulder to drop is a lateral shift of the rib cage to the other side. Feel this for yourself by relaxing your shoulders, letting them rest on the thorax, and then moving your rib cage to one side. Most of you will feel the unsupported shoulder fall away from your ear.

The shoulders can also shift anteriorly and posteriorly. We can also interpret this through the balance in the scapular 'X'. The pectoralis minor and serratus anterior will shorten in an anterior shift while the rhomboids and lower trapezius lengthen, and vice-versa with a posterior shift.

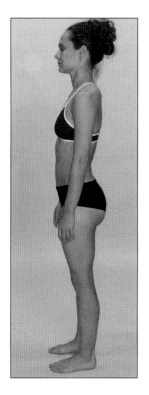 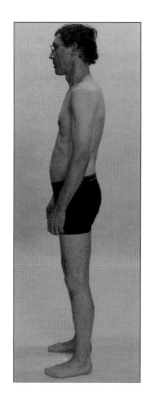 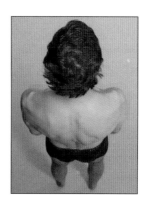

Figure 9.22a, b & c: To read anterior/posterior shifts we need to assess the relationship of the centers of gravity of the shoulder girdle and the rib cage. The center of gravity of the thoracic cage will be roughly halfway between the lower portion of the sternum and the spine, while the shoulder girdle can be seen as the midpoint of the 'V' created by the spine of the scapula and the clavicle. In our first model we see a good relationship between the two, but in the second we can clearly see the shoulder girdle has shifted forward from the center of gravity of the rib cage. This is especially apparent when we see the superior view and get another view of the 'V' between the two lines of bone.

The next axis of movement is rotation, when the scapula turns to face medially or laterally (the latter movement is restricted by the presence of the rib cage, so it is not often seen). The superior view of our second client (figure 9.22c) gives us an example of medially rotated scapulae. While this will often accompany an anteriorly shifted shoulder, it can also occur with a posterior shift, as seen in our third model (figure 9.23).

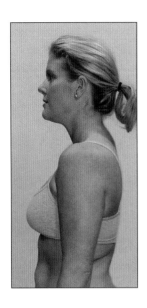

Figure 9.23: As we saw earlier, this model's shoulders are drawn back (posteriorly shifted) to counterbalance the weight of the head shifting forward and then medially rotated to facilitate the use of the arms in front of the body. If we are to satisfactorily ease the pattern of her shoulders, we will need to bring the head and neck in better alignment with the rib cage.

Our last axis of movement is tilt. This can be measured by looking at the angle at which the medial border lies relative to the ribs and spine. Tilting can occur in two planes: medial/lateral, which is a variation away from the parallel relationship the medial border of the scapula should have with the spine (presuming the spine to be straight enough, figure 9.24); and anterior/posterior, which is assessed by the angle between the scapula and the underlying ribs.

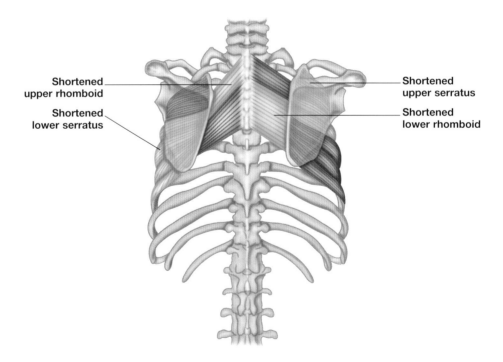

Figure 9.24: Medial/lateral tilt of scapula, otherwise referred to as upward/downward rotation, can be corrected by adjusting the different sections of the scapular 'X'.

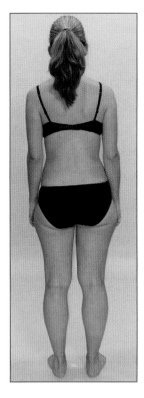

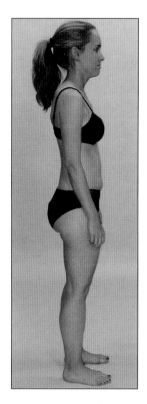

Figure 9.25: Here we can see a lateral tilt of both shoulders, as the lower portion of the medial borders are closer to the spine. So working the lower rhomboids and upper serratus anterior may be beneficial.

Figure 9.26: In this model we see a slight anterior tilt of the scapula in standing, but we can also see that her rib cage is tilting posteriorly. If we correct her rib cage (you can tilt the book until her thorax is vertical), we will also need to do quite a bit of work on the front of the shoulder girdle (pectoralis minor) to correct it.

Shoulder and Arm Techniques

Pectoralis Major and Sternocostal Fascia (SFL and SFAL)

Standing to one side of the client, use the fingers or soft fist of the hand next to the client to lift the tissue from the fifth rib in a superior direction. You will be working on either side of the sternum. For some larger male clients, you may be able to use both fists at once. For female clients, you will need to use only two or three fingers, particularly as you pass below the central part of the bra (ensure that you explain exactly where you are going and why, gaining permisssion from the client before starting the technique).

Start from above the xiphoid process and aim the stroke toward the proximal attachment of the clavicle. Two or three strokes can cover the areas superficial to, alongside and slightly lateral to the sternum, depending on the width of the tool you are using. Although general lifting strokes are good, you will also find plenty to work with in the detail of the sternocostal joints just to each side of the sternum.

The stroke can be extended to include the clavicular portion of the pectoralis major by following the line inferior to the collarbone. Whilst both sides of the chest can be worked from the same side, it can be easier for your body mechanics to change sides to work across the body as you come out along this upper portion.

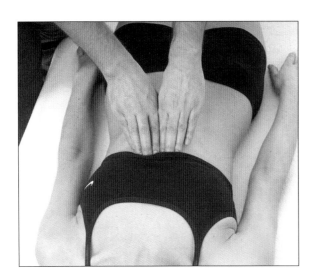 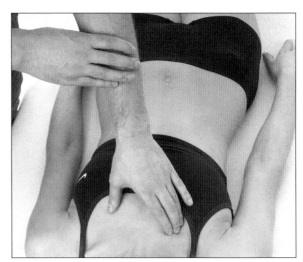

Figure 9.27a & b: Obtain permission from your client before lifting the fascia along and either side of the sternum and working out toward the humerus inferior to the clavicle.

Subclavius (DFAL)

The area below the clavicle can often be very restricted, particularly in anyone with breathing issues. To open this area more thoroughly and to gain direct access to the subclavius, roll your fingers under the bone and ask the client to externally rotate their arm. This will in turn rotate the clavicle away from your fingers.

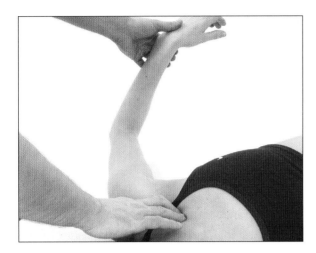
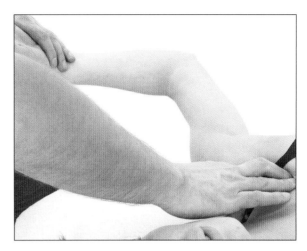

Figure 9.28a & b: Lock into the superficial tissue inferior to the clavicle and externally rotate the arm, to roll the clavicle to open the fascia and prepare the area for deeper work.

If the movement of the clavicle is restricted in the sternoclavicular joint, you may wish to work directly on the subclavius. To do this, bring your client near to you at the edge of the couch and have them reach up to the ceiling. Place your fingers inferiorly and deep to the bone, with the pads of the fingers against it. Then ask the client to slowly bring their elbow downward to the floor. The elbow should pass below the level of the edge of the couch in order to achieve a release in the subclavius.

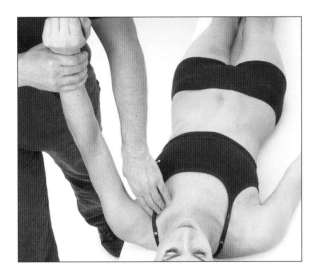
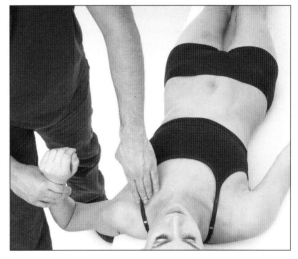

Figure 9.29a & b: With the arm raised, lock into the subclavius and then slowly horizontally abduct the arm toward the floor.

Pectoralis Minor

When working on this sensitive area we prefer to kneel or sit to the side of the client, allowing greater stability and therefore more relaxed hands as we enter an often challenging area for clients. Once again it is best to explain where you are going and why, and ask your client to alert you to any nerve sensations, as it is easy to impinge or stretch the fascia around the brachial plexus as you ease through the tissue. Should this happen, it is simply a case of retracting slightly and repositioning, maybe taking a slightly different angle to your approach. Try not to retreat completely or panic if it does happen. Coming in and out of the tissue too many times can be distracting to the client, as is any look of distress on your face.

The pectoralis minor is one of the main stabilizers of the shoulder girdle. It is an antagonist to the lower portion of the trapezius muscle, and has (at least) three slightly different directions of pull on the scapula, depending on the number of attachments it has to the rib cage. It is also enveloped within the clavipectoral fascia, which helps support the passage of the brachial plexus as it passes out and down the arm.

Seated or kneeling at roughly waist level on your client, glide the fingers of the 'head' hand deep to the lateral edge of pectoralis major, your fingertips gliding along, i.e. parallel to, not poking into) the ribs. Push your fingers from your shoulder; keeping your fingers as relaxed as possible allows the client and their tissue to open more easily, preventing guarding of the area.

The other hand supports the arm by holding at the wrist, having the arm slightly abducted to allow access, and can then guide the client into either one of two movements. Once the appropriate fibers of the pectoralis minor have been engaged, the client can then either bring their arm over their head, similar to swimming a very slow backstroke, or use their lower trapezius to bring their shoulder toward the midline and down their back. This latter movement can help with the retraining of the often weakened, under-used section of trapezius, while the former is more of a straightforward pin and stretch. Both movements can be altered in order to focus the stretch on the tissue along whichever section is the more restricted. For example, if the scapula is more medially rotated, then the upper (third rib) slip of pectoralis minor will be shorter, and retraction of the scapula emphasized. If the scapula is more anteriorly tilted, we need to focus more on the lower (fifth rib) slip by asking for more downward movement as we lock the tissue.

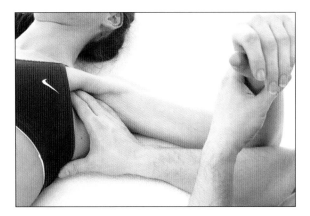 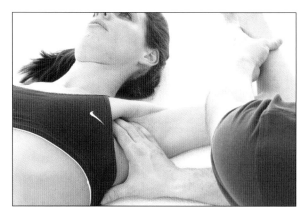

Figure 9.30a & b: Gliding between the back of pectoralis major and the rib cage, gently open the clavipectoral fascia to access and lock onto the pectoralis minor. Then either have the client reach back with their arm (as shown) or ask them to draw their shoulder-blades together and down their back to stretch.

Latissimus Dorsi and Teres Major – Scapulohumeral Freedom

Quite often the humerus and scapula can become quite tied together either because of, or possibly causing, shortness of the fascia around the posterior axilla. This can be checked by simply fully abducting the humerus and watching and/or feeling for the amount of scapular movement with humeral abduction. Should any restriction exist, simply relax the tissue a little by adducting the arm slightly. Sink into the myofascia of the latissimus dorsi and teres major which form the posterior wall of the axilla, and taking care not to stretch the skin, passively or actively abduct the arm over the client's head.

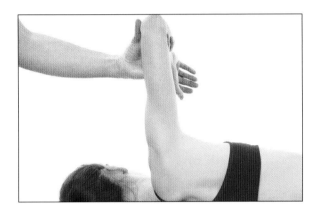 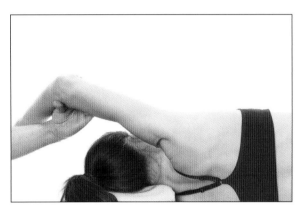

Figure 9.31a & b: With the client in side-lying, assess the relationship between the trunk and the proximal humerus. Feel for tight or restricted lines that tilt the scapula earlier than necessary.

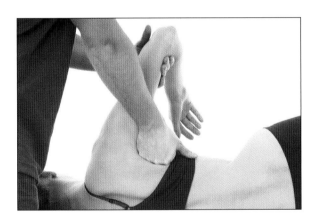 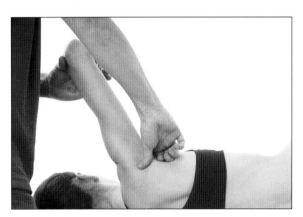

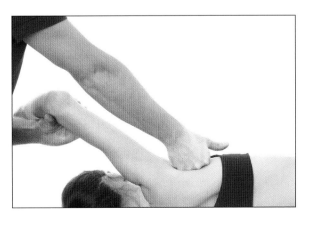

Figure 9.32a, b & c: With the arm relaxed lock into the tight lines with either a soft fist or knuckles, and then slowly abduct the humerus to stretch the tissue.

Just as with the hip joint, the glenohumeral joint is surrounded by a series of fan-shaped muscles or sequences of muscles that form a triangular pattern. From the near-horizontal fibers of infraspinatus to the near-vertical fibers of the lateral latissimus dorsi, we have a wide range of possible vectors of pull. Where the horizontal fibers will restrict the horizontal adduction above, the more vertical fibers of the latissimus dorsi will affect simple abduction of the arm (i.e. bringing the arm out to the side of the body and alongside the ear).

This movement can be assessed in standing and both passively and actively in side-lying. As you work, the angle of the client's arm movement can be altered to match that of the fibers of your target area: the more vertical the fiber, the more the arm can move toward the ear; to release the horizontal fibers, it will be more effective to reach the client's arm across the front of the body. These last two movements can easily be combined into one smooth sequence by simply altering the angles and position of your engagement and the direction of humeral movement. As with all these techniques, sensitive adjustment to the client's tissue pattern is more important than a rote recapitulation of our generalized descriptions.

Seated Latissimus Dorsi Release (SFAL)

With your client on the bench, engage the latissimus dorsi along the lateral aspect of the rib cage and ask your client to lift their arms out, up and forward. You will be able to isolate particularly tight areas by combining different variations of these movements.

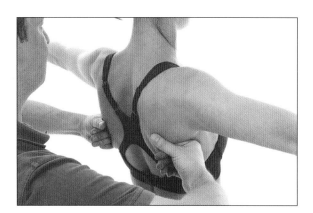
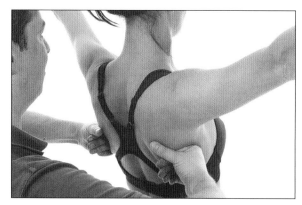
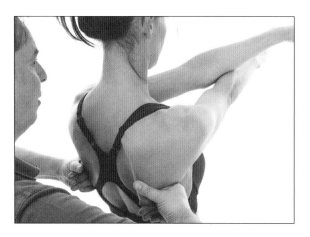

Figure 9.33a, b & c: Locking into the latissimus dorsi and teres major and having your client move their arms through a wide range of movement can help free the humerus from the scapula and trunk.

Rhomboids (DBAL)

In all but the military-type posture, the rhomboids are more likely to be locked long than too short, but they can vary in their length between the superior and inferior fibers. If we accept that the medial border of the scapula should be parallel to the spine in a neutral position, then if the scapula is tilting laterally the lower fibers of this muscle will be locked shorter relative to the superior fibers. The reverse will, of course, be true if the scapula is medially tilted (figure 9.24).

To isolate the sections of the rhomboids, work from the opposite side of the table and lock into the appropriate section, starting laterally to the spinous processes anywhere between C7 and T5, depending on which fibers are shortest, and moving toward the medial border of the scapula. In order to open the upper sections, ask the client to reach down to their foot as you glide out from the spine. For the lower portions, ask them to bring their arm out to the side and alongside their head. These two movements will open the upper and lower portions of the rhomboids respectively.

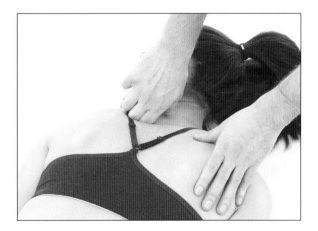 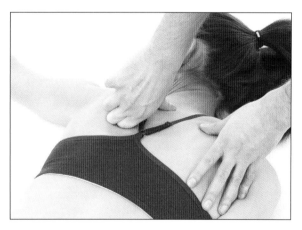

Figure 9.34a & b: To isolate the upper fibers, ask the client to reach down to their thigh as you work. To open the lower portion, have them reach their arm out to the side. This can be used to help reverse any medial or lateral tilt of the scapula.

Work transversely across the fibers in the case of any locked long myofascia. The rhomboids can be easily accessed from the head of the table, using a soft fist or elbow working down the body.

Serratus Anterior (SPL)

This extension of the rhomboids muscle can be more easily accessed with the client in either the side-lying or seated positions. It is a confusing muscle with many different fiber directions and so, like many others, will have to be worked in different directions, depending on the shoulder girdle position.

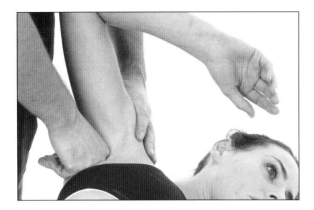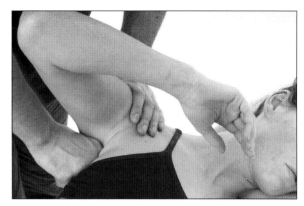

Figure 9.35a & b: Lightly engage the lateral border of the scapula with your proximal knuckles, taking care not to press onto either the ribs or the edge of the bone. Draw the scapula posteriorly, controlling and guiding the movement with the other hand cupped around the acromion process. When the tissue is engaged it can be stretched further by having the client draw their inhalation to the lateral ribs.

The upper fibers of serratus anterior are almost horizontal, pulling the scapula forward and round the thorax, while the lower fibers will draw it down inferiorly, laterally, and ultimately forward around the rib cage.

With the client in side-lying, use the proximal knuckles of your 'foot' hand gently along the lateral border of the scapula. The 'head' hand can encompass the acromion process, and between the two hands you will have almost complete control of the shoulder girdle. By taking the scapula posteriorly and superiorly, you can isolate the stretch into the lower fibers. Bringing these two bones straight back toward you will focus the movement on the middle or upper fibers. As you play with this movement, you can become quite precise and subtle in the identification of restricted lines. The movement is obtained by holding the scapula posteriorly as the client inhales. Ask the client to 'breathe up to my hand' in order to further emphasize the expansion of the rib cage.

When seated, you can work on both sides simultaneously, using the proximal knuckles to retract both scapulae, and then having the client inhale. This time the breath will be 'up and into the sternum, letting it lift'. The client can increase the stretch by holding their arms straight out in front and crossing them like scissors while you hold the scapulae in place. If one side is more restricted than the other, use one hand as a steadying hand while the other does the major work. Make sure that your arms are kept wide with the elbows elevated, the fists almost cleaving the scapulae off the thorax (but not squeezing the ribs). The same slight changes in angle of force can help fine-tune your direction onto the appropriate fibers.

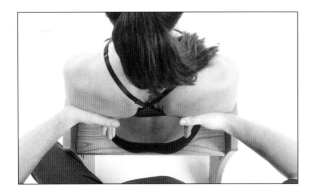

Figure 9.36: Kneeling behind the seated client, engage the lateral borders of both scapulae and draw them posteriorly around the rib cage. Then ask the client to breathe up into their sternum to open both serratus anterior.

Trapezius (SBAL)

Many references divide the trapezius into two (upper and lower) or three (upper, middle and lower) sections. We prefer to think of it as having four sections, as the anterior portion that attaches to the lateral third of the clavicle has a quite different function from the rest. It passes from the front to the back of the body, so it can pull the head forward as well as rotate it to the opposite side.

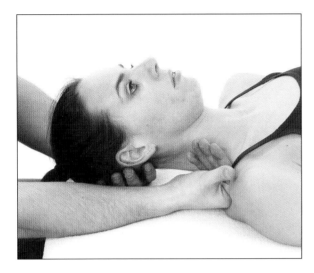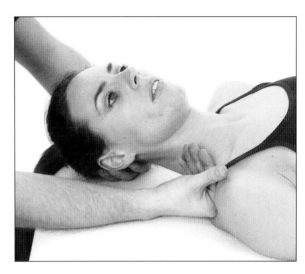

Figure 9.37: Use a soft fist to lock the tissue and glide the client's head into lateral flexion. Rotation and/or flexion can be added to gain extra precision of the technique.

Have the client supine to work with this anterior portion. Place one hand under the occiput to guide the movement and the other in a soft fist slightly anterior to the crest of the shoulder (you should easily palpate the anterior border of the trapezius; your contact should remain posterior to this edge). After you sink into the superficial and thin tissue of the trapezius, the client can then either actively or passively turn their head to the same side and glide it to the opposite side (ipsilateral rotation and contralateral side flexion) as you either glide along the fibers, opposing the movement, or lock in one place.

The upper portion of the posterior trapezius can be worked from the same position by bringing your contact posterior to the crest of the shoulder. Simply side flexing the head (actively or passively, but preferably actively) to the opposite side will help open it up.

The middle and lower sections will have to be accessed with the client in a prone, side-lying or seated position. Similar to the rhomboids, they are rarely locked short, and so more often require transverse strokes to release the fascia within the lengthened fibers. This can most easily be achieved with the client in a prone position as they reach forward (middle fibers) or overhead (lower fibers).

Rotator Cuff Techniques

External Rotators – Infraspinatus and Teres Minor (DBAL)

While your client is lying prone, have them move closer to the edge of the table to have their forearm hanging over the side, their elbow resting comfortably on the edge. Ask your client to keep their elbow in place but slowly bring the palm of their hand toward the ceiling. This will create an internal rotation of the arm to stretch the target tissue, as you are locked in the two muscles inferior to the spine of the scapula.

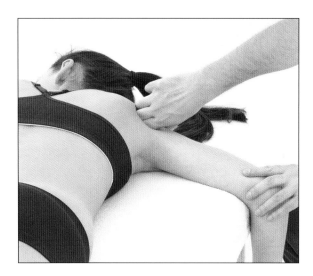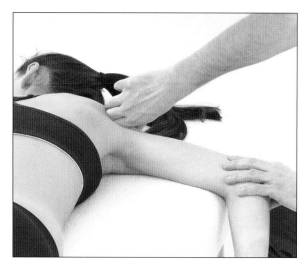

Figure 9.38a & b: Use your knuckles to lock into the infraspinatus and teres minor, and then have your client internally rotate their arm by lifting the palm of their hand toward the ceiling. Repeat this movement a few times as you engage into slightly different sections of the small fan of myofascia on the back of the scapula, while encouraging the medial rotation of the shoulder girdles. Be thorough, as this area is quite often locked short.

Internal Rotator – Subscapularis (DBAL)

There are certain areas in the body that get little attention, as they are hidden from view and protected from touch. The subscapularis is one of these, and we need to be aware of minimizing the discomfort as we approach it. Kneel or sit beside the client to ensure you have a stable base. Attempting this movement from standing can require extra tension in your body to stabilize. This can transfer into your contact, making these techniques more challenging to the client than they need to be.

To engage this muscle on the anterior (deep) surface of the scapula, it is easier to have the client bring their shoulder girdle onto your hand rather than vice-versa.

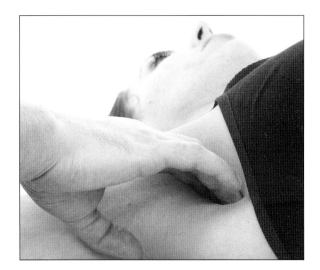

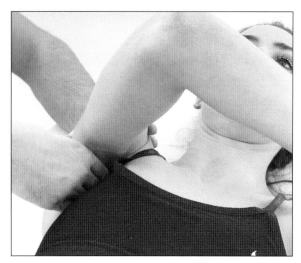

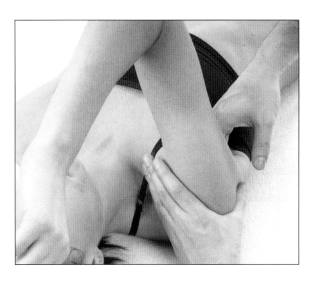

Figure 9.39a, b & c: Lightly sink your fingers into the septum between the anterior aspect of the scapula and the rib cage, opening the septum between the serratus anterior and subscapularis. Have the client reach across their body to bring the anterior aspect of the scapula (and therefore the subscapularis) onto your fingertips. Increase the pressure for the engagement by pushing on the acromion with your other hand. The client can then slowly externally rotate their arm to stretch.

Place your 'foot' hand on the side of the rib cage just anterior to the lateral border of the scapula. The 'head' hand can then come onto and guide the acromion process, as you ask the client to bring their shoulder forward and across their body. This will bring the scapula around and over your fingers.

Rather than pushing up and in with your fingers to engage the tissue, push the client's scapula onto your fingers by pressing gently down on the acromion with your 'head' hand. This way your working fingers can be as relaxed as possible as they engage the fascia over the subscapularis. Once you are securely locked in the tissue, ask the client to laterally rotate their arm with the elbow held close to the trunk, to bring the back of their hand toward you. Have them move their shoulder and practice the arm rotation before you start.

Abductor – Supraspinatus (DBAL)

The supraspinatus is a thick muscle lying deep to the trapezius in the trough above the spine of the scapula. It passes deep to the acromion above the head of the humerus to attach laterally, holding the humeral ball down into the joint and creating an abducting force on the arm.

The client can be prone, supine or side-lying, and have their arm slightly abducted to shorten the muscle as you sink into it sensitively but quite deeply and with an engagement to draw the tissue medially as they slowly adduct their elbow. Thumbs are probably the best tool to fit into the space, but try with your knuckles first in order to save your thumbs for more sensitive work.

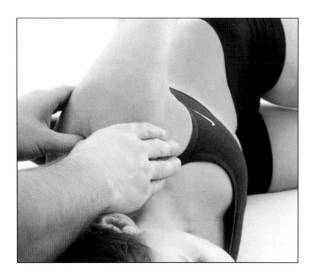 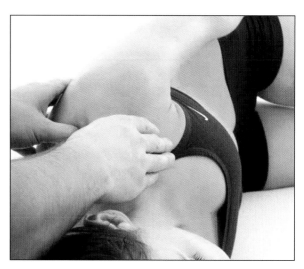

Figure 9.40a & b: Have the client in side-lying with their elbow pointing to the ceiling and abducted, to allow you to sink deeply into the supraspinous fossa. Then ask them to slowly glide their hand down their thigh to challenge the tissue.

External Rotators in Side-Lying – Infraspinatus and Teres Minor (DBAL)

Have a look at the relationship between your client's humerus and scapula as they move their arm from horizontal abduction to horizontal flexion (or simply ask them to reach forward) and assess how early in the movement the scapula starts to come with the arm. If the arm is 'tied' to the scapula by the external rotators, this restriction can encourage further medial rotation of the entire shoulder girdle. Releasing this area is therefore essential to gain lasting results from your work to re-situate the upper girdles.

Have the client in side-lying with their upper arm horizontally abducted. The knuckles of your 'foot' hand can engage the tissue of the infraspinatus and teres minor, while the 'head' hand supports the scapula at the acromion. The index finger of this upper hand can act as a fulcrum to encourage the movement to occur at the glenohumeral joint, as the client brings their arm across their chest.

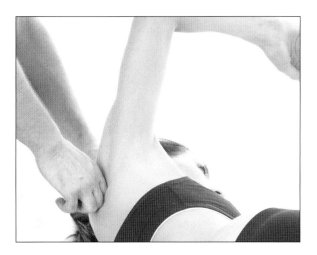
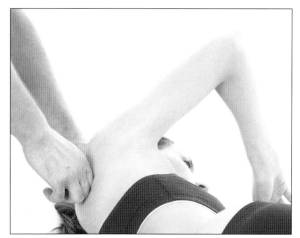

Figure 9.41a & b: Engage the teres minor and infraspinatus medially as the client reaches across the front of their body.

Opening the Flexor Compartment

The finger and wrist flexors are often overused and can be prone to extra stress because of an unsupported shoulder girdle. Common dysfunctions in this area are golfer's elbow and carpal tunnel syndrome. Both can benefit from this local work, but often require a balance that can be achieved all the way back to the rib cage and pelvis.

Have the client supine with their hand over the edge of the couch, the forearm supported on it, and then engage the flexor compartment with a soft fist, fingers or even an elbow. In cases of tendonitis at the proximal attachment we recommend working toward the elbow so as not to further stress the tissue. The reverse direction could be more relieving for carpal tunnel symptoms, and for those clients who seem to have extra flexion in their fingers. The client can flex and extend their wrist. You can ask for radial and ulnar deviation, or simply have them circle their hand as you work.

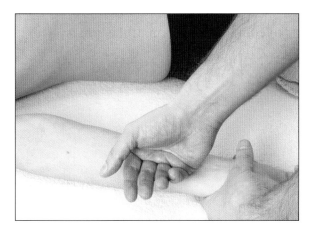
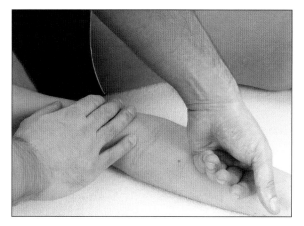

Figure 9.42a & b: Sink into the tissue of the flexors with either a soft fist or forearm and glide proximally or distally to open it, as the client flexes and extends their wrist and fingers.

Opening the Extensor Compartment

The extensors are much less sensitive than the flexors and can usually cope with the stronger contact of the forearm or elbow. The client positioning and movements are the same as for the flexors above. The extensors are more involved with tennis elbow, inflammation at their proximal attachment. Again, for long-term relief, you should work to achieve maximum support for the whole shoulder girdle, along with any local work to relieve the symptoms.

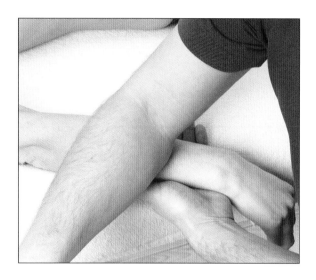

Figure 9.43: As with the flexors above, engage the tissue with whichever tool seems most appropriate and slowly draw the tissue proximally or distally, as the client moves their wrist and fingers.

Opening the Carpal Tunnel

The carpal tunnel is formed by a strong and tight retinaculum. This passes over an arch in the carpals, with the flexor tendons, blood vessels and nerves running underneath. A compartment-syndrome-type problem can arise when any of the tendons or their synovial sheaths become inflamed and swell to create an impingement on any of the other vessels. Some relief may be achieved by opening this fascial 'roof' of the tunnel.

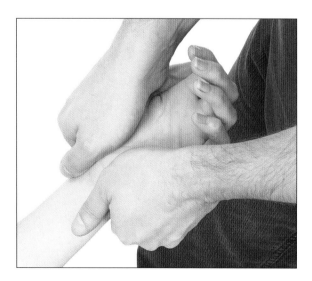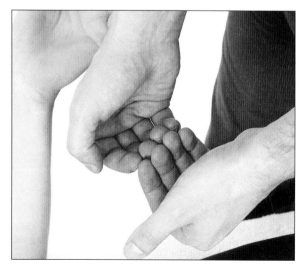

Figure 9.44a & b: Hold the wrist between your thenar eminence and fingers and push down and out with the base of your thumbs as you push up with your fingers, trying to open the front of the carpal tunnel.

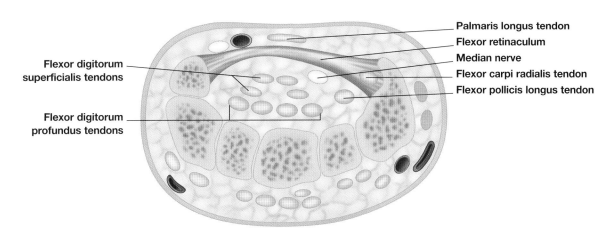

Figure 9.45: Cross-section of the wrist.

Use the thenar aspects of both hands to contact the lateral carpals, and then use your fingers on the dorsal aspect of the client's hand to push as you spread the front of the wrist with the base of your thumbs. Your intention is to open the front of the carpal tunnel, with the aim of stretching the fascial element of the carpal tunnel opening and giving more space for the underlying tendons.

Once again, though, you should pay attention to the rest of the shoulder complex, and make sure it is supported efficiently by the rib cage. Be sure to give any appropriate advice for aftercare and management. Care should also be taken in assessment, as many clients have been misdiagnosed as having carpal tunnel syndrome, when in fact the source of their problem is really the thoracic outlet and an impingement somewhere along its path. Learning some differential diagnostic skills or having a trusted colleague to refer to for a thorough diagnosis can therefore be especially useful in this area.

Unrolling the Sleeve

Many clients show a strong pattern of forearm pronation, which can appear as if their upper limb is medially rotated, the back of their hand presenting forward when standing. This will involve the pronator teres of the forearm but can also be helped by unwinding or unrolling the deep investing layer of antebrachial fascia. With the client supine, engage the tissue along the radial side and have the client supinate as you work across the forearm toward the ulna.

Occasionally clients can present with the opposite pattern, in which case it is a matter of simply working the posterior forearm as they turn into pronation.

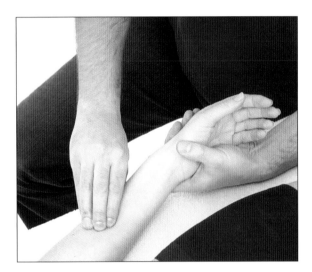 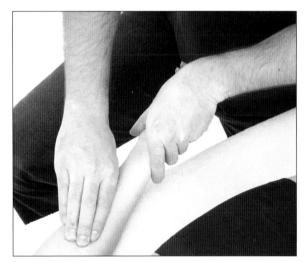

Figure 9.46a & b: With your fingers, work across the forearm as the client supinates and pronates their hand.

Releasing the Lateral and Medial Intermuscular Septa

The lateral and medial septa of the arm blend into the tendons of the wrist extensors and flexors respectively, and so working through these fascial areas can assist with releasing many held patterns along the Arm Lines. The lateral intermuscular septum is part of the Superficial Back Arm Line, and the Superficial Front Arm Line passes along the medial septum.

With the client supine (figure 9.47), use your fingers to access the fascial lines just slightly proximal to where they blend into the flexor and extensor tendons, and then have the client flex and extend their elbow as you spread the tissue.

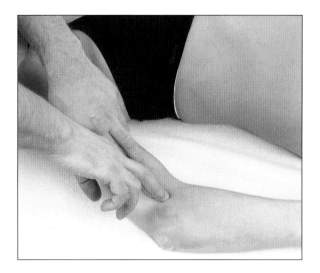
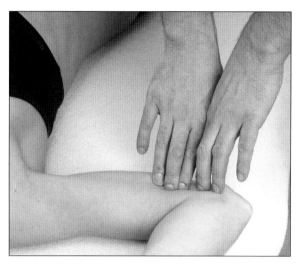

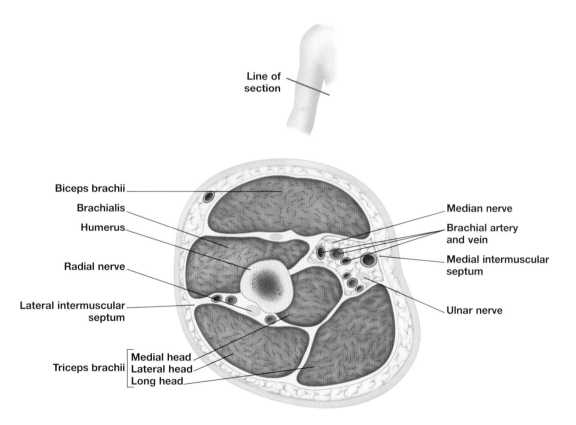

Figure 9.47a, b & c: Working with the lateral septa with the arm by the client's side. To access the medial septa, ask the client to abduct their arm and flex their elbow.

Releasing the Deltoid

Due to its triangular shape, the deltoid will be involved in both internally and externally rotated patterns of the humerus. Remember that, as it crosses only the glenohumeral joint, it will have little influence on the positioning of the shoulder girdle as a whole.

Place the client in side-lying and decide which aspect of the deltoid appears shorter. Have the client position their arm to shorten it. Engage into it, and then ask them to slowly perform the opposite movement, as shown in figure 9.49a & b.

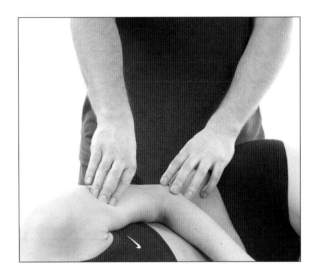
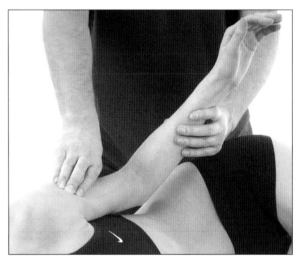

Figure 9.48a & b: Releasing the anterior deltoid as the client externally rotates.

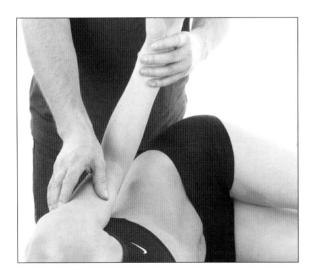
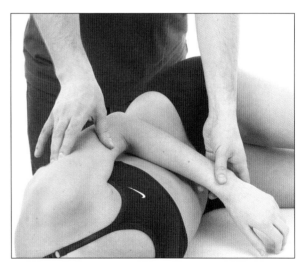

Figure 9.49a & b: Releasing the posterior deltoid as the client internally rotates.

Triceps Brachii

To release the superficial aspects of the triceps brachii, the client can be supine with their arm held upward, as you use your thumbs to lock into the tissue and resist the lengthening as the client flexes their elbow.

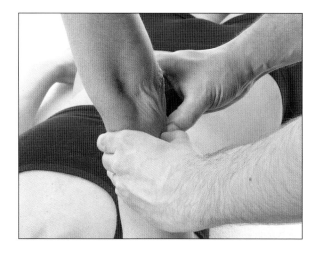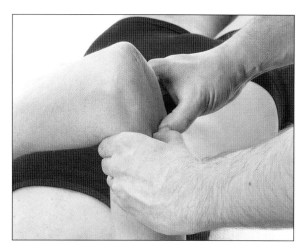

Figure 9.50a & b: Use your thumbs to engage the triceps brachii proximally, as the client flexes their elbow.

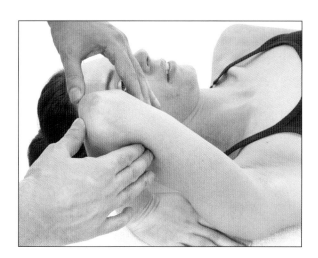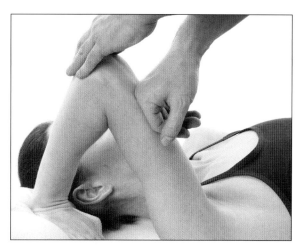

Figure 9.51a & b: With the client's hand resting on the table, or a bolster to the side of their head, engage the deeper aspect of the tissue between your fingers or the superficial aspect with a soft fist, as they reach away with their elbow and relax.

Another approach more likely to build tone in those concerned with hypotonic triceps 'wattles' involves an alternative position, which gives more flexibility in accessing the various aspects of the triceps brachii. Have the client place their hand on the table to the side of their head (a bolster can be used if their range of movement is not yet free enough, figure 9.51b). The deeper fibers can then be worked with the fingers from above, or the superficial aspect from beside the client using a soft fist. In this position the client's movement would be to reach up and back with their elbow. This will help open the back of the glenohumeral joint, releasing the long head of the triceps brachii.

Coracobrachialis

The coracobrachialis is an often-ignored muscle, but as an adductor of the arms it can be responsible for many restricted patterns. This occurs most obviously when the upper arm is held too close to the body, or when there is limited arm movement when walking. It can often be quite locked for ladies with larger chests who use their arms to stabilize or limit the movement of the breasts, particularly when running or engaged in other sports.

To find the coracobrachialis, place the fingers of one hand on the inside of the upper arm and ask the client to adduct their arm as you resist with your other hand at their elbow. They can then relax as you sink into the myofascia. Then ask them to reach their arm toward their feet, as you help draw the tissue down and out by curling your fingers through the muscle belly.

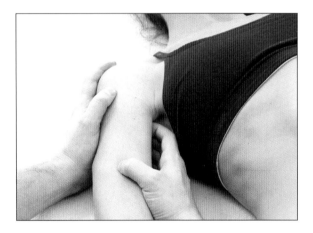 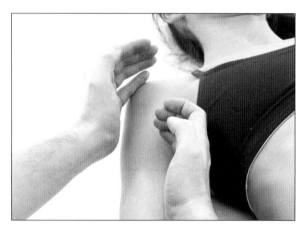

Figure 9.52a & b: The fingers of the working hand curl into the tissue of the coracobrachialis and draw it down as the client reaches their arm down along the table.

Biceps Brachii

The biceps brachii will obviously be shortened in those people with chronically flexed elbows – those who look as though they are constantly ready to draw a gun from their holster. A simple pin and stretch can open all of the superficial tissue of the front of the arm. The client lies with the elbow flexed as the therapist engages along the biceps brachii, and then the elbow is slowly extended.

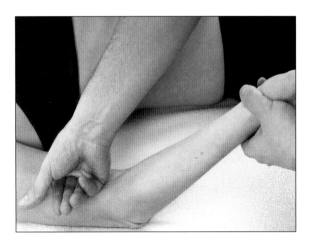

Figure 9.53: Locking into the tissue on the front of the arm with the elbow flexed and then slowly lengthening it.

Brachialis

Whilst much release can be attained through working the superficial tissue, always remember to look for any deeper muscles particularly single-joint muscles, as they are often more involved with the holding of a pattern, leaving the superficial structures freer for movement. The elbow flexors are a case in point, where much of the pattern can be held by the brachialis. To be more specific for this tissue, use your fingers either side of the biceps brachii tendon and sink inward and upward to resist the lengthening of the tissue as the client extends their arm.

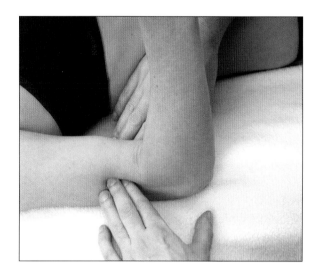

Figure 9.54: To engage the deeper elbow flexors use your fingers to engage below the biceps brachii and into the myofascia around the brachialis.

Integration

We have endeavoured, within the confines mandated by a book, to set down a reasonably complete set of techniques for approaching structural balance via the myofascia. Some areas, for reasons of endangerment or anatomical complexity, we have left for a future volume of advanced techniques. Other manual therapies – for articular tissues via thrusting or unwinding, for the cranial or visceral cavities – are certainly congruent with ours, but beyond the scope of this book.

Movement training methods, from yoga to Pilates to athletic training, are also very useful for promoting structural balance by way of neuromuscular strength and coordination (as well as encouraging fascial equilibrium) and can often be considered in tandem with this approach. We hope you have found these pages helpful, but we are well aware that the ideas contained within form only part of human balance.

We have said it often, but we will repeat it here, that to be presented, techniques must be broken down and shown in a linear fashion. In practice, we hope you will feel free to adapt them for your own body and for particular clients who require some modification. Practice is the one sure way to smooth out the rough edges and to build efficiency and flow into your application of this method.

No technique is good in itself; it must serve wholeness to have value. Develop your visual assessment skills to integrate a series of techniques into a coherent session, they must form part of a larger context to better serve the client.

BodyReading accurately allows you to follow not the book but the client's body – the ultimate authority – in the journey toward full function. For those who learn better via video, most of these techniques and others are available through our websites and other educational outlets in the manual field. Our classes, offered around the world, provide the best access to confident application of these skills; this book is designed as an aide-mémoire for students, but we know it will also serve some people who cannot come to such classes.

If you have reached this page, you are surely interested in making life less effortful and more pain free for other people. We wish you good luck and good skill in this worthy task.

James Earls & Thomas Myers

Appendix 1: The Anatomy Trains Lines

Individual myofascial meridians can be viewed as one-dimensional tensional lines that pass from attachment point to attachment point and from one end to the other. They can be viewed as two-dimensional fascial planes that encompass larger areas of superficial fasciae. Or they can be seen, as they are here, as three-dimensional set of muscles and connective tissues, which, taken together, comprise the entire volume of the musculoskeletal system.

Summary of the Lines

With these rules in mind, we can construct twelve myofascial meridians in common use in human stance and movement:

• Superficial Front Line
• Superficial Back Line
• Lateral Line (2 sides)
• Spiral Line
• Arm Lines (4)
• Functional Lines (2 – front and back)
• Deep Front Line

The first three lines are termed the 'cardinal' lines, in that they run more or less straight up and down the body in the four cardinal directions – front, back, and left and right sides.

Superficial Front Line

The Superficial Front Line (SFL) runs on both the right and left sides of the body from the top of the foot to the skull, including the muscles and associated fascia of the anterior compartment of the shin, the quadriceps, the rectus abdominis, sternal fascia, and sternocleidomastoideus muscle up onto the galea aponeurotica of the skull. In terms of muscles and tensional forces, the SFL runs in two pieces – toes to pelvis, and pelvis to head, which function as one piece when the hip is extended, as in standing (see figure 1).

In the SFL, fast-twitch muscle fibers predominate. The SFL functions in movement to flex the trunk and hips, to extend the knee, and to dorsiflex the foot. In standing posture, the SFL flexes the lower neck but hyperextends the upper neck. Posturally, the SFL also maintains knee and ankle extension, protects the soft organs of the ventral cavity, and provides tensile support to lift those parts of the skeleton which extend forward of the gravity line – the pubes, the ribcage, and the face. And, of course, it provides a balance to the pull of the Superficial Back Line.

A common human response to shock or attack, the startle response, can be seen as a shortening of the SFL. Chronic contraction of this line – common after trauma, for example – creates many postural pain patterns, pulling the front down and straining the back.

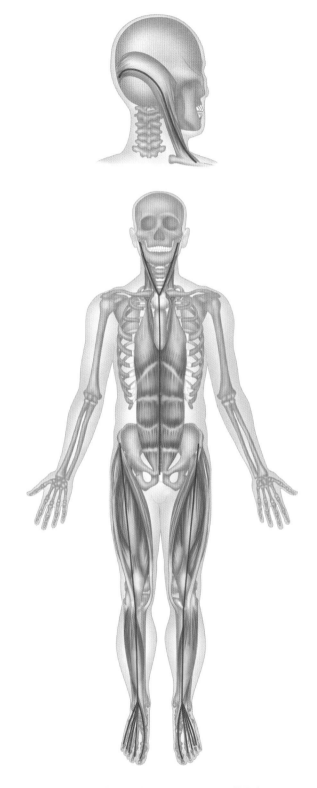

Figure 1: The Superficial Front Line (SFL).

Superficial Back Line

The Superficial Back Line (SBL) runs from the bottom of the toes around the heel and up the back of the body, crossing over the head to its terminus at the frontal ridge at the eyebrows. Like the SFL, it also has two pieces, toes to knees and knees to head, which function as one when the knee is extended. It includes the plantar tissues, the triceps surae, the hamstrings and sacrotuberous ligament, the erector spinae, and the epicranial fascia.

The SBL functions in movement to extend the spine and hips, but to flex the knee and ankle. The SBL lifts the baby's eyes from primary embryological flexion, progressively lifting the body to standing (see figure 2).

Posturally, the SBL maintains the body in standing, spanning the series of primary and secondary curves of the skeleton (including the cranium and heel in the catalogue of primary curves, and knee and foot arches in the list of secondary curves). This results in a more densely fascial line than the SFL, with strong bands in the legs and spine, and a predominance of slow-twitch fibers in the muscular portion.

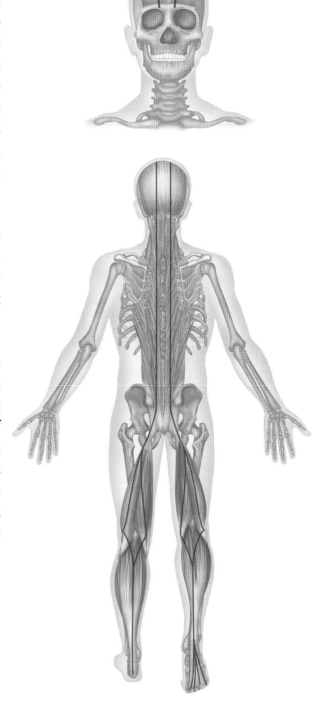

Figure 2: The Superficial Back Line (SBL).

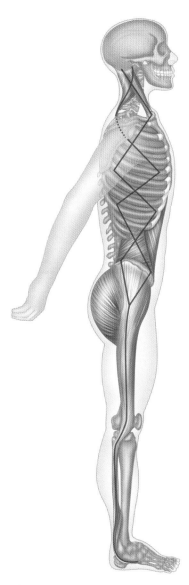

Figure 3: The Lateral Line (LTL).

Lateral Line

The Lateral Line (LTL) traverses each side of the body from the medial and lateral midpoints of the foot around the fibular malleolus and up the lateral aspects of the leg and thigh, passing along the trunk in a woven pattern that extends to the skull's mastoid process (see figure 3).

In movement, the LTL creates lateral flexion in the spine, abduction at the hip, and eversion at the foot, and also operates as an adjustable 'brake' for lateral and rotational movements of the trunk.

The LTL acts posturally like tent guywires to balance the left and right sides of the body. Also in human movement, the LTL contains movement more than creates it, directing the flexion-extension that characterizes our direction through the world, restricting side-to-side movement that would otherwise be energetically wasteful.

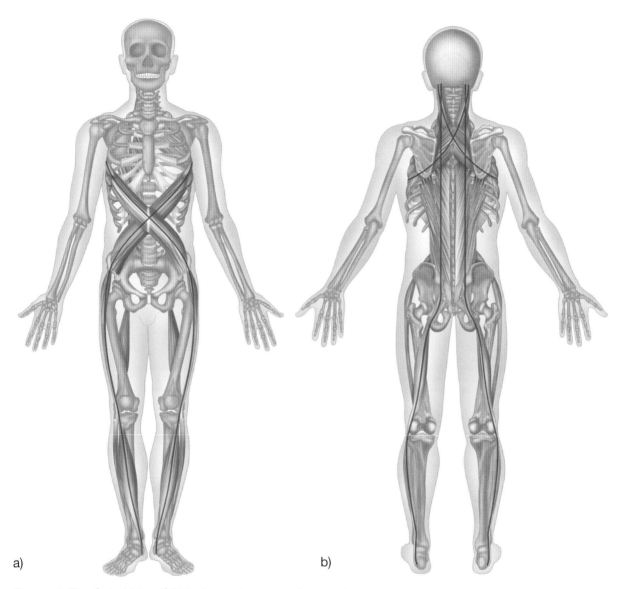

Figure 4: The Spiral Line (SPL); a) anterior view, b) posterior view.

Spiral Line

The Spiral Line (SPL) winds through the three cardinal lines, looping around the trunk in a helix, with another loop in the legs from hip to arch and back again. It joins one side of the skull across the midline of the back to the opposite shoulder, and then across the front of the torso to the same side hip, knee and foot arch returning up the back of the body to the head (see figure 4).

In movement, the SPL creates and mediates rotations in the body. The SPL interacts with the other cardinal lines in a multiplicity of functions.

In posture, the SPL wraps the torso in a double helix that helps to maintain spinal length and balance in all planes. The SPL connects the foot arches with tracking of the knee and pelvic position. The SPL often compensates for deeper rotations in the spine or pelvic core.

Arm Lines

- Superficial Front Arm Line (SFAL)
- Deep Front Arm Line (DFAL)
- Superficial Back Arm Line (SBAL)
- Deep Back Arm Line (DBAL)

The four Arm Lines run from the front and back of the axial torso to the tips of the fingers. They are named for their planar relation in the composition of the shoulder, and roughly parallel the four lines in the leg. These lines connect seamlessly into the other lines particularly the Lateral, Functional, Spiral, and Superficial Front Lines (see figure 5).

In movement the arm lines place the hand in appropriate positions for the task before us – examining, manipulating, or responding to the environment. The Arm Lines act across ten or more levels of joints in the arm to bring objects to us or to push them away, to push, pull, or stabilize our own bodies, or simply to hold some part of the world still for our perusal or modification.

The Arm Lines affect posture indirectly, since they are not part of the structural column. Given the weight of the shoulders and arms, however, displacement of the shoulders in stillness or in movement will affect other lines. Conversely, structural displacement of the trunk in turn affects the arms' effectiveness in specific tasks and may predispose them to injury.

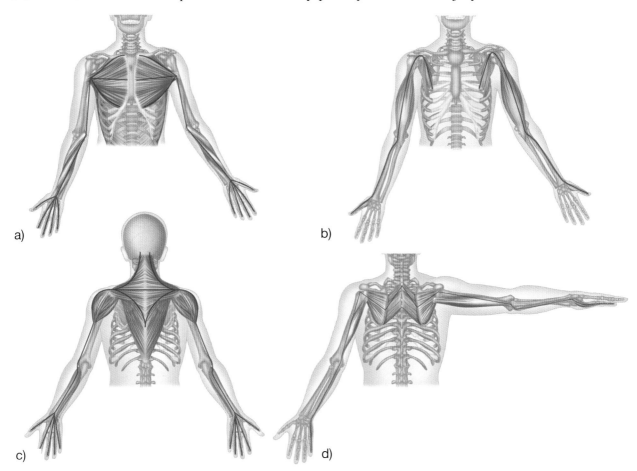

Figure 5: The four Arm Lines; a) Superficial Front Arm Line, b) Deep Front Arm Line, c) Superficial Back Arm Line, d) Deep Back Arm Line.

Beyond the straightforward progression of the meridians from the trunk to the four corners of the hands, there are many 'crossover' muscles that link these lines to each other, providing additional support and stability for the extra mobility the arms have relative to the legs.

Functional Lines

- Front Functional Line (FFL)
- Back Functional Line (BFL)

The two Functional Lines join the contralateral girdles across the front and back of the body, running from one humerus to the opposite femur and vice-versa (see figure 6).

The Functional Lines are used in innumerable movements, from walking to the most extreme sports. They act to extend the levers of the arms to the opposite leg as in a kayak paddle, a baseball throw or a cricket pitch (or vice-versa in the case of a football kick). Like the Spiral Line, the Functional Lines are helical, and thus help create strong rotational movement. Their postural function is minimal.

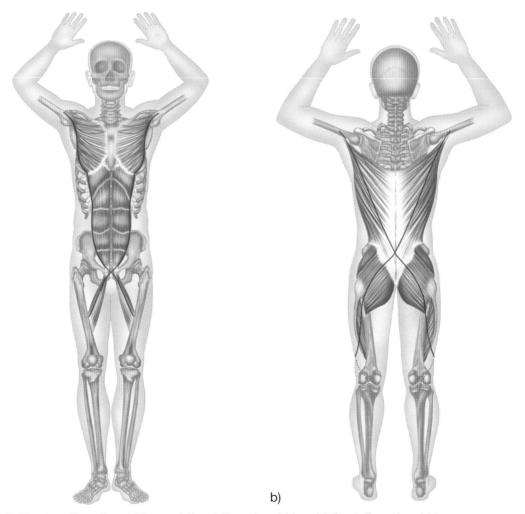

a)   b)

Figure 6: The two Functional Lines; a) Front Functional Line, b) Back Functional Line.

Deep Front Line

The Deep Front Line (DFL) forms a complex core volume from the inner arch of the foot, up the inseam of the leg, into the pelvis and up the front of the spine to the bottom of the skull and the jaw. This 'core' line lies between the Front and Back Lines in the sagittal plane, between the two Lateral Lines coronally, and is wrapped circumferentially by the Spiral and Functional Lines. This line contains many of the more obscure supporting muscles of our anatomy, and because of its internal position has the greatest fascial density of any of the lines (see figure 7).

Structurally, this line has an intimate connection with the arches, the hip joint, lumbar support, and neck balance. Functionally, it connects the ebb and flow of breathing (dictated by the diaphragm) to the rhythm of walking (organized by the psoas). In the trunk, the DFL is intimately linked with the autonomic ganglia, and thus uniquely involved in the sympathetic-parasympathetic balance between our neuro-motor 'chassis' and the ancient organs of cell-support in the ventral cavity.

The importance of the DFL to posture, movement, and attitude cannot be over-emphasized. A dimensional understanding of the DFL is necessary for successful application of nearly any method of manual or movement therapy. Because many of the movement functions of the DFL are redundant to the superficial lines, dysfunction within the DFL can be barely visible in the outset, but these dysfunctions will gradually lead to larger problems. Restoration of proper DFL functioning is by far the best preventive measure for structural and movement therapies.

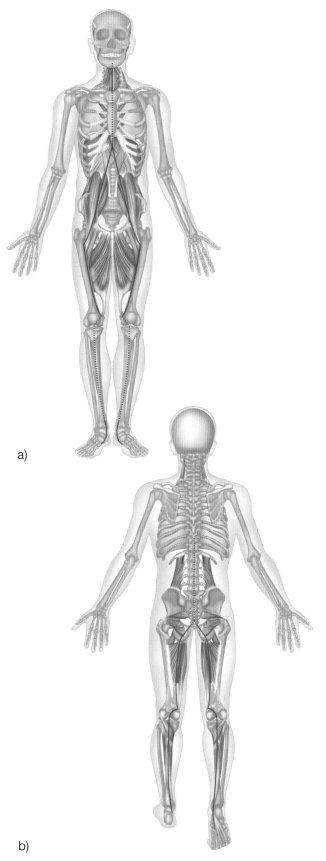

a)

b)

*Figure 7: The Deep Front Line (DFL);
a) anterior view, b) posterior view.*

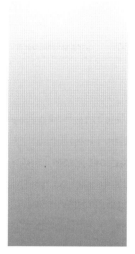

Appendix 2: Contraindications

The techniques and ideas portrayed within this text are safe for the majority of clients when applied by manual therapists with a solid understanding of the body. There are of course conditions under which these techniques should not be applied, or should at least be modified to suit the needs of the client.

It is important to understand the implications of your touch for the client. This can be mechanical, physiological, psychological or spiritual and will vary according to your own style of practice and the constitution of the client. The deeper your knowledge of underlying pathologies and the biological and psychological effects of fascial release technique the better able you will be to adapt these techniques in appropriate ways.

Common sense can guide you through most of the local contraindications and help you decide when to avoid a certain area. Cuts, wounds, broken bones and bruises, skin rashes or cracked eczema (to name a few) may not respond well to strong work. Working away from these areas with the rest of the body will often be useful to reduce any compensations to areas of pain or restriction. You may need to pay more attention to positioning and structural support of your client as you work.

The idea of providing a list of conditions indicating when to adapt or to omit treatment has some use but is ultimately limited and will be different for practitioners from various backgrounds. What may be a caution for one practitioner may be a contraindication for another and could possibly be an indication to apply the work for a third.

When to apply this work is often a question of the depth and style of your training background. If you are conversant, for example, with spondylolisthesis, then the ideas contained in this book may be usefully adapted to support the client. If you are running for the medical dictionary or have no clear picture of the anatomy involved, then it is perhaps best to leave these clients for another practitioner.

With these provisos, we have chosen to include some useful guidelines for contraindications, with thanks to Dr. Schleip for his permission to adapt his work, with the caution that you stay inside the boundaries of your own professional training. If you are ever in doubt about the implications of this style of treatment for your client, seek further advice from an experienced colleague or from the client's medical practitioner. These days there are many Internet forums and online references that can also be valuable sources of information.

Working to change structure via the fascia can require a lot of energy from the client. Certain conditions may impede the client's ability to process the therapeutic input, so be careful with people with challenges such as fibromyalgia, chronic fatigue syndrome and Epstein-Barr-type diagnoses or symptoms. The work can be useful, particularly to resolve breathing issues, but may need to be adapted to shorter and lighter input.

Similarly, older clients may require an adapted approach depending on their energy level and tissue health. If osteoporosis is an issue then structural change may be best achieved slowly to allow for the change in mechanics to remodel the trabeculae to the new pattern over a period of months rather than days and weeks. Any large fast changes will alter the pathway the forces take through the bones, and if there has been insufficient time for bone remodeling the bones are effectively weakened.

Any potential weakness (diagnosed or suspected) of the bones will also need to be taken into consideration when applying pressure techniques.

There are many conditions that are coming into the bodywork realm that may be considered specialisms. Previously contraindicated clinical presentations can now be considered for treatment if the practitioner is informed of the surrounding implications. Bodywork during and after cancer care is one such example. There are now numerous references and training workshops focusing on the issues to be considered.

The presence of cancer has often been listed as a contraindication in order to protect the therapist in case the cancer spreads and the bodyworker is blamed because of the effects on circulation.

Similarly, providing bodywork to pregnant women has often been advised against due to the potential of miscarriage or premature birth. In both cases (and we are by no means implying pregnancy to be a medical condition) caution must be applied and the body respected, but intelligently applied bodywork can be very helpful in supporting the client.

Deep abdominal work should of course be avoided with pregnant (or potentially pregnant) women. As the pregnancy progresses the body will be experiencing many preparatory but also compensatory changes that the practitioner can aid and ease. The time to work for longer lasting change, however, will be in the post-partum period.

Other areas may include neurological and psychological conditions, all of which again may be **contraindicated or indicated depending on the therapist's level of training or other areas of expertise.**

Arteriosclerosis: This is hardening of the arteries. Care is needed because there is usually some atherosclerosis and high blood pressure associated with this. No bodywork in advanced stages. Get medical clearance for your work if the client takes medication for circulatory problems. Aspirin and other blood-thinning medications (like warfarin and heparin) significantly increase the risk of bruising in the tissues.

Atherosclerosis: This is a build-up of plaque in artery walls. Care needs to be taken so that any thrombi are not dislodged. (See under 'Embolism or thrombus')

Autoimmune diseases: The immune system produces antibodies against the body's own tissues. Do not work on acutely inflamed tissues.

a) Lupus – The immune system attacks the connective tissue mainly in the skin, kidneys, joints and heart. Contraindicated during acute flares.

b) Rheumatoid arthritis – The immune system attacks the joints and their associated muscles, tendons, ligaments and blood vessels. Contraindicated during inflammatory stage. (Note: with osteoarthritis, deep bodywork tends to be more successful).

c) Scleroderma ("hardened skin") – This is manifested by a build-up of collagen fibers around the organs (which can lead to problems with absorption when the build-up is around the small intestines) and in the dermis of the skin, as well as an increasing stiffness at the joints, along with muscle weakness. Contraindicated during inflammatory phase.

d) Ankylosing spondylitis – An inflammation of tissues around the spine causes the connective tissues of the sacrum and spine to solidify. Don't work on areas of pain and inflammation in acute episodes.

Bipolar disorder (manic depression): During a manic phase, deep bodywork could be contraindicated, since it could then increase the amplitude of the extreme mood swings.

Borderline psychological diagnosis: Be careful with clients on the border between neurosis and full psychosis. There have been a (very) few reports about deep work triggering a psychotic episode. Full psychosis is in most cases a contraindication, and of course should be performed with supervision by a psychiatrist.

Cancer: Connective tissue can often act as a barrier to the spread of cancer by encapsulating the cancerous cells. Deep work could theoretically cause the cancerous cells to metastasize (move through the circulatory or lymphatic system to other places in the body). In fact, most cancers have been shown not to metastasize in this fashion, but Non-Hodgkin's lymphoma may be an exception to this rule, and this work is thus contraindicated for this condition. This work is usually no problem if the person has had a clean bill of health for five years. Pay special attention to lumps in the abdomen, or lymph nodes in the groin or the armpit. (Lumps in the abdomen could be hard faeces. Let the client monitor it: if there is no change after three days, suggest to the client that further investigation might be a good idea.)

After mastectomy, check with the doctor as to whether massage in the area (including the arm) is indicated. Sometimes it is not advisable to increase the lymphatic flow in that area.

Where axillary or inguinal lymph nodes have been removed for staging purposes – or where lymph nodes have been cleared or irradiated – the lymphatic system in the affected quadrant remains compromised. Any intervention that might stimulate circulation in the affected quadrant (i.e., deep pressure, vigorous massage, heat application, etc.) can lead to the development of lymphoedema or worsen lymphoedematous swelling where it already exists.

Cerebral palsy: A study on cerebral palsy and Rolfing® found that in mild and moderate cases, Rolfing® (a form of fascial release work) may be helpful; in serious cases, function might get worse. In the most recent scientific information, connective tissue restrictions are a more important factor in CP patients than was previously thought (e.g., tissue shortness in the triceps surae often limits walking ability because of very limited dorsiflexion and mobility of the feet).

Connective tissue disease: This includes diseases such as osteomyelitis, lupus and scleroderma. Do not perform deep work.

Diabetes: Be careful about tissue condition and loss of sensation. Don't do deep work on the area of recent insulin injection as this could accelerate insulin uptake. Beware of bruising, which is facilitated in these people.

Embolism or thrombus:

a) Venous emboli usually lodge in the lungs, causing pulmonary embolism.

b) Arterial emboli can lodge in the coronary arteries, causing a heart attack; in the brain, causing a stroke; in the kidneys; or in the legs, leading to phlebitis.

In the case of thrombosis, deep bodywork is usually contraindicated because of the risk of dislodging a thrombus. If the client takes blood thinners as a medical precaution against clotting, ask for a medical clearance for any kind of deep tissue work affecting the circulatory system. This precaution is even more strongly advocated in clients who have had a pulmonary embolus, or have had a Greenfield filter installed (a filter in the vena cava to prevent blood clots from reaching the lungs).

Epilepsy: avoid hyperventilation. Avoid this work all together if the client is restricted from exercise.

Headaches: Some types of headaches get worse with any kind of bodywork around the head, neck and shoulder area. This is quite common for migraines in the acute stage, probably due to infection and/or central nervous system (CNS) overstimulation. If the client has previous experience with receiving massage as a remedial treatment, they can often tell whether it is helpful or not to work on their upper body. Tension headaches (which are usually more bilateral) tend to respond more positively.

Heart conditions: It is generally all right to work on clients who have heart conditions if they are not restricted from exercise (if their fingernails get purple or blue, stay off).

Hemangioma: This is a congenital benign tumor, made up of newly formed blood vessels. There are different types, usually on the skin, yet sometimes also in the brain and viscera. Do not perform deep work in the abdominal area in cases of known visceral types (e.g., hepatic hemangioma) due to the severe danger of internal bleeding.

Herpes: Don't touch infected areas. This also applies to other potentially infectious skin conditions, including warts.

High blood pressure (extreme): Don't work in way that makes clients hold their breath. Deep work on clients with uncontrolled high blood pressure should be with medical supervision (deep bodywork often raises blood pressure).

Impaired elimination systems: Use caution with colostomies, candida and kidney and liver issues. Work carefully and leave more spacing between sessions.

Intervertebral disc problems: With non-acute cases, avoid shearing motions and extreme bending. Don't decompensate a stable system. With acute cases, although bodywork can help create space for the retreat of the tissue and resolve some of the secondary compensations, be very careful and don't work on the affected segment alone, since local muscle spasms may have developed there as an important protection for the weakened or herniated disc. Releasing this muscular bracing too soon may put the client in danger.

Intrauterine device (IUD): Be careful with any deep abdominal work in female clients who use an intrauterine device for birth control. It is possible that an IUD may become displaced, possibly leading to complications.

Menstruation: If the client tends to have very strong menstrual symptoms with high amounts of blood loss, any kind of deep tissue work or even massage in the area of the pelvis, abdomen and thighs – if done around the days of the client's period – can sometimes increase circulation and therefore the severity of the menstruation. Either give the client the option to cancel a session if the date coincides with a strong menstrual period, or give only a very gentle movement awareness session that does not tend to increase circulation in the pelvic region.

Neurological conditions: This work is contraindicated for any systemic inflammatory conditions of the nervous system, for example, chronic inflammatory demyelinating polyneuropathy (CIDP). Pain medication: Use caution regarding reduced sensation and greater possibility of tissue or nerve damage. (Same with paresthesia.)

Pregnancy: The general rule of thumb is no deep work. Be aware: the danger of triggering a miscarriage by strong myofascial work is greatest during the first three months (especially at around ten weeks, and particularly through work around the pelvis, abdomen, adductors, medial legs or feet). Later in pregnancy this gets less likely, though it is conceivable that stimulation of reflex points could start a premature delivery. If you work with somebody who is pregnant, you may want to have them sign a form that they are aware of the increased risks and still want to get deep work from you.

Working with pregnant women is a massage specialty, and those with more experience can work beyond these guidelines.

Septic foci: Avoid working with clients who have this condition, due to the possibility of spreading the infection.

Special nose conditions: Nasal work should be approached with caution in regular cocaine users and in cases of nasal polyps and reconstructive nose surgery.

Tooth Abscesses: Avoid intraoral work on clients with this condition.

Varicose veins: Avoid working with the affected veins.

Whiplash: If the affected area is inflamed, the condition might get worse with myofascial work.

Do not perform deep work with:

- **Aneurysm.**
- **Bone fractures or acute soft tissue injuries.** Wait for full healing, which can take six weeks to three months.
- **Cortisone treatments.** Wait two to three months.
- **Fever.**
- **Haemophilia.**
- **Hodgkin's disease** (cancer of lymph system).
- **Infectious conditions.** With some exceptions, like HIV: get medical supervision.
- **Inflammatory conditions, such as tendonitis and bursitis.** These are contraindicated during acute stages; work peripheral to the site is possible when inflammation has subsided.
- **Leaky gut syndrome.**
- **Leukemia.**
- **Osteoporosis.** This occurs usually in post-menopausal women.
- **Phlebitis.** The risks are the same as for embolism or thrombosis (see above).
- **Recent scar tissue (including regular or plastic surgeries).** Do not work on these areas until the scarring process is complete (usually at least six weeks after surgery).

Cautions

Unless you are legally licensed to practice healing:

1. Don't prescribe, not even vitamin C.
2. Never label or name any condition; don't diagnose (yet you can refer to a previous diagnosis of a medical doctor).
3. Be careful with people who are in psychotherapy or are seeing a doctor. (Their psychotherapist or physician should know they are getting bodywork.)

In General

Ask about the client's medical history (including medications) before work begins. If ever in doubt, get medical supervision.

Bibliography

Acland, R.D.: 1996. *Atlas of Human Anatomy (DVD)*. Lippincott, Williams & Wilkins, Baltimore

Agur, A.M.R. & Dalley, A.F.: 2004. *Grant's Atlas of Anatomy*. Lippincott, Williams & Wilkins, Baltimore

Albinus, B.S., Hale, B.R. & Coyle, T.: 1989. *Albinus on Anatomy*. Dover Publications, New York

Alexander, F. M.: 2001. *The Use of the Self*. Orion, London

Alexander, R. M.: 2010. *The Human Machine*. Columbia University Press, New York

Aston, J.: 1998. *Aston Postural Assessment Workbook: Skills for Observing and Evaluating Body Patterns*. The Psychological Corporation, San Antonio

Aston, J.: 2006. Lecture Notes

Barlow, W.: 1973. *The Alexander Technique*. Alfred A Knopf, New York

Barnes, J.F.: 1990. *Myofascial Release: A Comprehensive Evaluatory and Treatment Approach*. Myofascial Release Seminars, Paoli

Barral, J-P. & Mercier, P.: 2000. *Visceral Manipulation, Revised Edition*. Eastland Press, Seattle

Barral, J-P.: 2001. *Manual Thermal Diagnosis*. Eastland Press, Seattle

Becker, R.O. & Selden, G.: 1998. *The Body Electric*. Quill, New York

Beil, A.: 1997. *Trail Guide to the Body*. Books of Discovery, Boulder

Berman, M.: 1990. *Coming to Our Senses: Body and Spirit in the Hidden History of the West*. Bantam Books. New York

Bogduk.: 1992. From Bogduk et el Anatomy and biomechanics of psoas major. *Clinical Biomechanics*; 7:109–119

Bond, M.: 1997. *Balancing the Body: Self-help Approach to Rolfing Movement*. Inner Traditions, Rochester

Bonner, J.T.: 1990. *On Development: Biology of Form*. Harvard University Press, Cambridge, MA

Busquet, L.:1992. *Les Chaines Musculaire, Tome 1–IV, Freres, Mairlot, Maitres et Cles de la Posture*

Cailliet, R. & Fechner, L.G: 1996. *Soft Tissue Pain and Disability*. F.A. Davis Company, Philadelphia

Calais-Germain, B.: 1993. *Anatomy of Movement*. Eastland Press, Seattle

Chaitow, L.: 1980. *Soft Tissue Manipulation*. Thorsons, Wellingborough

Chaitow, L.: 1996. *Palpatory Skills*. Churchill Livingstone, Edinburgh

Chaitow, L. & Fritz, S.: 2006. *A Massage Therapist's Guide to Understanding, Locating and Treating Myofascial Trigger Points*. Churchill Livingstone, Edinburgh

Clemente, C.: 1987. *Anatomy: A Regional Atlas of the Human Body*, 3e. Lea & Febiger, PA

Cohen, B.B.: 1993. *Sensing, Feeling and Action*. North Atlantic Books, Berkeley

Cottingham, J.T. & Brown, M.: 1989. *Healing Through Touch: A History and a Review of the Physiological Evidence*. Rolf Institute, Boulder

Dart, R.: 1950. Voluntary musculature in the human body: the double-spiral arrangement. *British Journal of Physical Medicine*, 13 (12NS): 265–268

Darwin, C.: 1965. *The Expression of the Emotions in Man and Animals*. University of Chicago Press, Chicago

Dawkins, R.: 1990. *The Selfish Gene*. Oxford University Press, Oxford

Dawkins, R.: 2006. *The Blind Watchmaker*. W.B. Norton, New York

Dawkins, R.: 2006. *Climbing Mount Improbable*. W.B. Norton, New York

Ellenberger, W, et al.: 1966. *An Atlas of Animal Anatomy for Artists*. Dover Publications, New York

Fast, J.: 1970. *Body Language: the Essential Secrets of Non Verbal Communication*. MJF Books, New York

Feitis, R. (ed.): 1985. *Ida Rolf Talks About Rolfing and Physical Reality*. Rolf Institute, Boulder

Feitis, R. & Schultz, L.R. (eds.): 1996. *Remembering Ida Rolf*. North Atlantic Books, Berkeley

Feldenkrais, M.: 1994. *Body Awareness as Healing Therapy: the Case of Nora*. Harper & Row, New York

Feldenkrais, M.: 1991. *Awareness Through Movement: Easy-to-do Health Exercises to Improve Your Posture, Vision, Imagination and Personal Awareness*. Harper Collins, New York

Feldenkrais, M.: 2005. *Body & Mature Behavior: a Study of Anxiety, Sex, Gravitation and Learning*. North Atlantic Books, Berkeley

Fuller, R.B. & Applewhite, E.: 1982. *Synergetics: Exploration in the Geometry of Thinking*. Prentice Hall, New York

Fuller, B. & Marks, R.: 1973. *The Dymaxion World of Buckminster Fuller*. Anchor Books, New York

Gellhorn, E.: 1970. The emotions and the ergotropic and trophotropic systems. *Psychologische Forschicht*, 34: 48–94

Gershon, M.D.: 2001. *The Second Brain*. Harper Collins, New York

Gorman, D.: 2002. *The Body Moveable*. Ampersand Press, Toronto

Gray et al.: 1995. *Gray's Anatomy, 38e*. Churchill Livingstone, Edinburgh

Grey, A., Wilber, K. & McCormack, C.: 1990. *Sacred Mirrors*. Inner Traditions, Rochester, VT

Grundy, J.H.: 1982. *Human Structure and Shape*. Noble Books, Chilbolton, Hampshire

Hanna, T.: 1968. *Somatics: Reawakening the Mind's Control of Flexibility, Movement and Health*. Perseus Books, Jackson

Hanna, T.: 1993. *Body of Life: Creating New Pathways for Sensory Awareness and Fluid Movement*. Healing Arts Press, Rochester, VT

Hatch, F. & Maietta, L.: 1991. Role of kinesthesia in pre- and perinatal bonding. *Pre- & Peri-Natal Psychology*, 5(3), Spring 1991. Info: Touch in Parenting, Rt 9, Box 86HM, Santa Fe, NM 87505

Hildebrand, M. & Goslow, G.: 2001. *Analysis of Vertebrate Structure, 5e*. John Wiley & Sons, New York

Horwitz, A.: 1999. Integrins and health. *Scientific American*, January 52–59

Huijing, P.A.: 2009. Epimuscular myofascial force transmission between antagonistic and synergistic muscles can explain movement limitation in spastic paresis; article in *Fascia Research II: Basic Science and Implications for Conventional and Complementary Health Care*. Elsevier, Munich

Hungerford, M.: 1999. Lecture Notes

Ingber, D.: 1998. *The Architecture of Life*. Scientific American, January 48–57

Iyengar, B.K.S.: 2001. *Light on Yoga*. Thorsons, London

Johnson, D.: 1977. *The Protean Body: a Rolfer's View of Human Flexibility*. Harper Collins, New York

Kapandji, I.: 1982. *The Physiology of Joints, 5e, Vol. 1–3*. Churchill Livingstone, Edinburgh

Kendall, F. & McCreary, E.: 1983. *Muscles, Testing and Function, 3e*. Lipincott, Williams & Wilkins, Baltimore

Kessel, R.G. & Kardon, R.H.: 1979. *Tissues and Organs: Text Atlas of Scanning Electron Microscopy*. W.H. Freeman, San Francisco

Kurtz, R.: 1990. *Body Centered Psychotherapy: the Hakomi Method*. Liferhythms, Mendocino, CS

Juhan, D.: 1987. *Job's Body*. Station Hill Press, Tarrytown, New York

Latey, P.: 1979. *The Muscular Manifesto*. Private edition, UK

Latey, P.: 1997. Themes for therapists series. *J. of Bodywork and Movement Therapies,* 1: 44–52, 107–116, 163–172, 222–230, 270–279

Leonard, C..: 1998. *The Neuroscience of Human Movement*. Mosby, St. Louis, MO

Levine, P.: 1997. *Waking the Tiger: Healing Trauma – the Innate Capacity to Transform Overwhelming Experiences*. North Atlantic Books, Berkeley

Lockhart, R.: 1970. *Living Anatomy: a Photographic Atlas of Muscles in Action*. Faber & Faber, London

Lowen, A.: 2006. *The Language of the Body: Physical Dynamics of Character Structure*. Bioenergetics Press, Alachua

Maitland, J.: 1995. *Spacious Body*. North Atlantic Books, Berkeley

Mann, F.: 1974. *Acupuncture: the Ancient Art of Chinese Healing*. Random House, New York

Margules, L. & Sagan, D.: 1995. *What is Life?* Simon & Schuster, New York

Masters, R. & Houston, J.: 1978. *Listening to the Body: the Psychophysical Way to Health and Awareness*. Delacorte Press, New York

Maupin, E.: 2005. *A Dynamic Relation to Gravity Volume 1: the Elements of Structural Integration*. Dawn Eve Press.

McMinn, R.M.H., Hutchings, R.T., Pegington, J. & Abrahams, P.H.: 1993. *Color Atlas of Human Anataomy, 3e*. Mosby-Year Book, St. Louis

Milne, H.: 1998. *The Heart of Listening: Visionary Approach to Craniosacral Work, Volume 1*. North Atlantic Books, Berkeley

Mollier, S.: 1938. *Plastiche Anatomie*. J.F. Bergman, Munchen

Montagu, A.: 1987. *Touching: Human Significance of the Skin, 3e*. Harper & Row, New York

Morgan, E.: 1994. *The Descent of the Child: Human Evolution from a New Perspective*. OUP, Oxford

Morgan, E.: 1994. *Scars of Evolution: What Our Bodies Tell Us About Human Origins*. OUP, Oxford

Myers, T.: 2009. *Anatomy Trains, 2e*. Churchill Livingstone, Edinburgh

Myers, T.: 1999. *Body to the Third Power*. Self-published

Myers, T.: 1998–99. Kinesthetic dystonia. *J. of Bodywork and Movement Therapies,* 1998, 2(2) 101–114, 2(4), 231–247, and 1999, 3(1) 36–43, 3(2) 107–116

Myers, T.: 1997. The anatomy trains. *J. of Bodywork and Movement Therapies,* 1(2) & 1(3)

Nelson-Jones, R.: 2005. *Theory and Practice of Counselling 4e*. Sage, London

Netter, F.H.: 1989. *Atlas of Human Anatomy, 2e*. Icon Learning Systems, New Jersey

Noble, E.: 1993. *Primal Connections*. Simon & Schuster, New York

Oschman, J.L.: 1997. *Readings in the Scientific Basis of Bodywork*. NORA, Dover, NH

Oschman, J.L.: 2000. *Energy Medicine: the Scientific Basis*. Churchill Livingstone, Edinburgh

Pedrelli, A., Stecco, C. & Day, J. A. 2009. Treating patellar tendinopathy with Fascial Manipulation. *J. of Bodywork and Movement Therapies, Vol. 13,* Issue 1, Pages 73–80, Elsevier, Edinburgh

Pert, C.: 1997. *Molecules of Emotion: Why You Feel the Way You Feel*. Prentice Hall, New York

Platzer, W.: 1986. *Color Atlas and Textbook of Human Anatomy, 3e Revised, Volume 1*. Georg Thieme Verlag, Stuttgart

Polhemus, T. (ed.): 1978. *The Body Reader: Social Aspects of the Human Body*. Pantheon Books, New York

Preece, et al.: 2008. Variation in pelvic morphology may prevent the identification of anterior pelvic tilt. *J. of Manual & Manipulative Therapy,* 16(2): 113–117, Maney Publishing

Radinsky, L.B.: 1987. *The Evolution of Vertebrate Design*. Chicago University Press, Chicago

Reich, W.: 1949. *Character Analysis*. Simon & Schuster, New York

Rolf, I. P.: 1977. *Rolfing*. Healing Arts Press, Rochester, VT

Rolf, I.P.: 1978. *Ida Rolf Talks About Rolfing and Physical Reality*. Rolf Institute, Boulder, CO

Romer, A. & Parsons, T.S.: 1986. *The Vertebrate Body, 6e*. Thomson Learning, New York

Schleip, R.: 1992. *Talking to Fascia, Changing the Brain*. Rolf Institute, Boulder, CO

Schleip, R.: 2003. Fascial plasticity – a new neurobiological explanation: parts 1 & 2. *J. of Bodywork and Movement Therapies,* Jan, 7(1) 11–19 and Apr, 7(2) 104–116, Elsevier, Edinburgh

Schultz, L. & Feitis, R.: 1996. *The Endless Web*. North Atlantic Books, Berkeley

Schwind, P.: 2006. *Fascial and Membrane Technique: A Manual for Comprehensive Treatment of the Connective Tissue System*. Churchill Livingstone, Edinburgh

Simons, D., Travell, J. & Simons, L.: 1998. *Myofascial Pain and Dysfunction: the Trigger Point Manual, Vol. 1*. Lippincott, William & Wilkins, Baltimore

Singer, C.: 1957. *A Short History of Anatomy & Physiology From the Greeks to Harvey*. Dover, New York

Smith, F.F.: 1989. *Inner Bridges: A Guide to Energy Movement and Body Structure*. Humanics New Age, Atlanta, GA

Smith, J.: 1998. *Shaping Life*. Yale University Press, New Haven, CT

Schneider, G.: 1975. *Fasciae: Applied Anatomy & Physiology*. Kirksville College of Osteopathy, Kirksville, MO

Stecco, C. et al.: 2008. Histological study of the deep fasciae of the limbs. *J. of Bodywork and Movement Therapies, Vol. 12,* Issue 3, Pages 225–230. Elsevier, Edinburgh

Still, A.T.: 1910. *Osteopathy: Research and Practice*. The Journal Printing Co., Kirksville, MO

Stirk, J.: 1988. *Structural Fitness*. Elm Tree Books, London

Sultan, J.: 1986. *Toward a structural logic: the internal-external model notes on structural integration*, 86:12–18 (Available from Dr. Hans Flury, Badenerstr 21, 8004 Zurich CH)

Sweigard, L.: 1998. *Human Ideokinetic Function*. University Press of America, New York

Talbot, M.: 1996. *The Holographic Universe*. Harper Collins, New York

Thompson, D.W.: 2009. *On Growth and Form: the Complete Revised Edition*. Dover Publications, New York

Todd, M.E.: 1937. *The Thinking Body: Study of the Balancing Forces of Dynamic Man*. Princeton Book Co., New York

Travell, J.G. & Simons, D.G.: 1999. *Myofascial Pain and Dysfunction: The Trigger Point Manual, Vol. 1: Upper Half of Body, 2e*. Williams & Wilkins, Baltimore, USA

Travell, J.G. & Simons, D.G.: 1999. *Myofascial Pain and Dysfunction: The Trigger Point Manual, Vol. 2: The Lower Extremities*. Williams & Wilkins, Baltimore, USA

van der Wal, J.: 2009. The architecture of the connective tissue in the musculoskeletal system – an often overlooked functional parameter as to proprioception in the locomotor apparatus. *International Journal of Therapeutic Massage & Bodywork: Research, Education & Practice, Vol 2, No.4*. American Massage Therapy Association

Vander, A. et al.: 1990. *Human Physiology, 5e*. McGraw-Hill, New York

Varela, F. & Frenk, S.: 1987. The organ of shape. *J. of Social Biological Structure*, 10:73–83

Werner, R.: 2008. *A Massage Therapist's Guide to Pathology, 4e*. Lippincott, Williams & Wilkins, Baltimore

Whitfield, P.: 1995. *From So Simple a Beginning: the Book of Evolution*. Macmillan, New York

Resources

There are a number of resources available from Kinesis to supplement and further speed your learning, some of which are listed below, and all of which may be ordered on-line. A number of workshops are also available worldwide exploring fascial anatomy, the Anatomy Trains, BodyReading and Fascial Release Technique. If you are interested in putting all of this information into a stronger context, then you may also be interested in our Structural Integration program (Kinesis Myofascial Integration) that combines the work of Dr. Rolf with Thomas Myer's work on the Anatomy Trains lines to provide a comprehensive framework for working in spatial medicine.

Further information on all of our courses, workshops and available product is available from the websites below.

Anatomy Trains book
The text maps out a 'longitudinal' myofascial anatomy, showing how the muscles are linked in series through the fascial webbing. The second edition includes numerous updates including important new findings in recent fascial research, photographs of the Anatomy Trains myofascial meridians dissected, new appendices on Structural Integration protocols based on the Anatomy Trains concept, and a comparison of the myofascial meridians with the meridians of acupuncture.

BodyReading 101™
A 3-DVD set, which can be used as a workbook, containing both tutorial and case histories. With more than 30 practice clients for standing posture and 12 for gait analysis, plus sections on assessing breathing and sitting, the 3-DVD set lets you test your own growing understanding before getting Thomas Myer's 'expert' opinion with his experienced eye.

Anatomy Trains Revealed: Dissecting the Myofascial Meridians
A 3-DVD set using real-time classroom video and photographs, which presents an unfolding first-hand voyage of discovery in the field of manual and movement therapies – a unique 21st century view of fascial anatomy in manual and movement therapy unexplored from the first dissections in the Renaissance until now.

Anatomy Trains DVDs
A 10-DVD set, which contains both theory and anatomy of the lines and technique tutorials. Fascial Plane and Fascial Release Techniques are presented as an integrated series for each of the Anatomy Trains lines. Currently there are eight technique based DVDs, which illustrate Chapters' 3 through 9 of the book respectively. The other two DVDs cover an introduction to Fascia Tensegrity and give an overview of the anatomy of the Lines. Each DVD is 1.25 hrs long and is credited under Category A for the NCBTMB. Tom demonstrates the techniques in a small-class, mentoring-type situation, with the student's questions, Tom's corrections, and client feedback all contributing to your being able to apply these techniques with ease and confidence.

Anatomist's Corner
A collection of articles by Tom Myers that appeared in *Massage and Bodywork* from 2000 to 2005. This 204-page spiral bound book has full color illustrations and 29 articles on such topics as **History of Anatomical Concepts, The Cell and Fascia, Structural Bodywork, Anatomy Unbound, The Psoas Series and The Anatomy of Energy.**

These and many more items are available from www.anatomytrains.co.uk (European orders) or www.anatomytrains.com (rest of the world)

Fascial Release Wax
A specially formulated medium to allow grip into the tissue and still provide a small amount of lubrication for gliding with the techniques is available from www.songbirdnaturals.co.uk

Other Useful Resources

www.somatics.de
A comprehensive listing of both research and general articles on fascia for practitioners and others who may be interested.

www.deeptissuemasagemanual.com
This is the home page of Art Riggs, talented practitioner and teacher. He offers great resources for more information on Fascial Release Technique and various aspects of practice including a very interesting monthly newsletter.

www.fasciaresearch.de
Stay up to date with the Fascia Research Project at the University of Ulm, Germany, home to Dr. Robert Schleip and a team of other pioneers in the field.

www.theiasi.org
The International Association of Structural Integrators® gives various listings of further education courses, Structural Integration trainings and practitioners.

Index

Index of Muscles